Virginia Art

Anne E Watmough

chipmunkapublishing
the mental health publisher

Anne E Watmough

Published by
Chipmunkapublishing
United Kingdom

http://www.chipmunkapublishing.com

Copyright © 2016 Anne E Watmough

ISBN   978-1-78382-257-7

Chapter 1 THE ASSAULT

It is a June summers day and I am outside sitting in my fragrant smelling garden. The weather is warm but rain is now threatening and I will have to go indoors soon.

My late husband Mark was a gardener by profession and with what he taught me and since his death I have made myself a beautiful garden. I find my solitude and peace there and it is an ongoing work of love. It is a place to escape from the realities and unrealities of my life.

I now live alone except with my lovely cat for company. He is pure love and no messing and I feel I am lucky to have him.

At present I am in the process of attempting a meeting with a hospital manager, to be accompanied by an advocate, with a complaint to the hospital about my treatment that I received whilst a patient there. It occurred when I was kept in solitary, known as the area of High Dependency.

I am looking for, at the most, a written apology. When I refused my medication, believing that my life was in danger, I was forced onto a bed and my knickers were pulled down and I was injected against my will into each buttock. Once with Lorazepam and once with Haldol, which are anti-psychotics. This happened three times and by two male nurses and three females.

I was prescribed by my psychiatrist tablets of Haldol, Lorazepam and Valium 2mg three times daily and I felt so awful physically I knew my life had to be in danger. So I refused to take the tablets. Then they injected me and I realized afterwards that the injections, because of the way I was feeling, were probably a purer form of the medication. So I told them they could continue to inject me but I would not take the tablets. I was then 60 years old and was quite aware of what was happening to me and what they were doing.

During Christmas 2011 whilst I was in solitary, two men in uniform who looked like armed guards came into my room and said I had to go with them immediately. So I dressed quickly in what clothes I could find and with no underwear on, my pyjama top and wearing damp jeans they whipped up my belongings, some of which had been soaking in the sink, and whisked me into a state of the art security vehicle.

They took me from Shelton Psychiatric Hospital in Shrewsbury to The Priory, Cheadle Hulme in Stockport, Manchester. Where I became a patient from Stokesay Ward onto the Pankhurst Unit.

This happened around the time I was applying to go to tribunal to contest my Section 3 of the Mental Health Act 1983, which I was detained under at the time.

Reaching Stockport was kind of like returning home, because my mother was raised there and it was where she grew up. She used to take us by bus to visit my aunty and Granny every Xmas when we would all receive presents.

My Granny and aunty lived in the house where my mum grew up with her 11 sisters and brothers in the area of Reddish. Although I never was given access to walk the grounds during my months stay on the Pankhurst Unit I felt close to the area which used to be home.

Pankhurst Unit was not unlike a high security prison and not what you would expect a hospital to be like. You might be asking yourself what my particular crime was? Was I a danger to myself or the public? My crime? I became overwhelmed with fear and I called the police out on numerous occasions, because I relate police to protection being a law abiding citizen.

I thought I was being stalked online and that somebody or some people were going to harm me and my son. I couldn't figure out why anyone would stalk me because although I access radical feminist websites and buy books on this and psychiatric books I am nothing at all special. There was no threatening emails just an intuition and feeling I was being watched online. No evidence at all. Just the odd thing would happen to alert my suspicion. It so pointed to my craziness but I know it is real.

I was exchanging emails with Ginger Breggin and sometimes I felt that certain ones I had posted to her she was not receiving. So one Saturday afternoon I sat down and checked. It took me two hours of actually sorting which had been sent and which she had responded to and in fact the ones that were most important to me she did not receive.

Also I could not get any messages posted on the comments pages of any feminist website. I posted comments on around five websites and none got onto their pages. I asked my son and brother and they said this was quite normal. That thousands of people comment and send messages and sometimes they do not get received because of faults in the system. But my suspicions were alerted. Simply because on one website titled RadFem the prominent article writer FCM in her private box says she does not respond to strangers but your message may or may not get through to me. And I felt that none of them were. Because one was actually printed on their page. Its contents were about the second movement which I was involved with in the 1970's and a feminist elite Kameraderie commented beneath it and thanked FCM for drawing her attention to this Strong Original Thinker. Which was me! So this threw me. Why just one comment printed if what I was saying was worth reading?

I had to put it down to there being a perfectly sound reason and explanation for what was happening to me on line. Ginger Breggin probably didn't want to comment on my emails. And the feminist sites were overwhelmed with emails and although mine was recognized they really hadn't time for me. But I still felt I was being watched.

Then the land line phone I was using went down. It was really strange because I had two lines with BT on the same phone. I had a line for broadband and line just for calls. And the line I could use for calls and call out on went down. The line for broadband was alright. There was nothing wrong with the equipment and the operator at BT spent three hours trying to help but she couldn't. There seemed nothing wrong with the line or the equipment itself. I just couldn't call out on my phone.

When Lee became manic I was beside myself with worry. I kept calling the police on the phone and asking for their help. The police leered at me on the other end of the phone when I said I thought my son was really ill and needed help getting into hospital. I just had my mobile then to call 999 if I needed help. I felt as though someone meant me and my son harm. In fact I felt as though we could be abducted. I became extremely paranoid and pulled the telephone socket off the wall. I was seeking help because Lee was vulnerable and yes in danger because later at one time I had callers pretending to be police but who weren't. I had called the police out and these men turned up dressed in uniform but without radios. And one was chatting me up and the other asked for my telephone number. What eventually happened was that a policeman dislocated my sons arm and he was in plaster for three months, so I had every right to be concerned.

So I thought maybe there would be something I had written in my journals that could give the chief of Dyfedd Powys police an idea who should want to do this to us. I placed them in a box and on the Monday morning I took my mobile to call for a taxi into town and it went haywire. The screen just simply scrambled. And I couldn't call out. I became terrified then because I knew I had lost all of my life lines. So I put it in the box with my journals and letter to the chief of police and went to a neighbours to ask her to call a taxi for me which she did. I was going to post the box at the post office and needed some money so I went into my local bank. A car pulled up outside which I could see through the window and I panicked thinking this was a threat. I pushed the box over the counter and told the assistant to give it to the police then I left. She thought it was a bomb.

I went to the post office and bought some survival stuff which I thought might come in handy if I was abducted and then dumped in the middle of nowhere because I live in a rural area and it was the middle of winter. I bought stuff like a plastic table cloth to keep me dry somewhere if I needed to sleep outdoors or in a damp partially sheltered place and chocolate which every soldier has packed in her rations.

I got a taxi home packed a survival bag and went round to my son's flat and he wasn't there so I asked a neighbour if she would call out the police once again as I actually feared something awful had happened to him. He had been arrested for disturbing the peace at a pub in town. I found out later that the police had shoved his arm so violently up his back they had dislocated it. But I didn't know then about the criminals who pretend to be police. So, in some respects my feelings were justified. Then they arrived and took me to the station where I was interviewed by a social worker, psychiatrist and GP. And admitted. But nobody told me anything about what happened to my son.

So my crime? Wasting police time. This warranted a two month detention in a psychiatric Unit.

My son and I were patients in the same hospital. He was on the male admittance ward where my husband had passed away two years earlier and I was on the female admittance ward opposite. I didn't see him during that time and they whisked him away to a hospital in Stafford. Then me to The Priory in Cheadle Hulme.

When I arrived at The Priory the doctor there said I was under his care because they 'Simply didn't know what to do with me!' I had become a problem to them. Not because I was violent to staff or other patients but because I had the whole situation weighed up and I knew I could in fact die because of the toxic chemicals they were forcing into me. I have witnessed other people die in front of my eyes due to adverse affects caused by these toxic medications. And I am aware of much worse. Like the brain damage called Tardive Dysconisea that is caused by these anti-psychotics.

There was one particular young nurse who was very verbally abusive towards me. She wasn't just down right rude she was aggressive and verbally aggressive towards me. Before she left after driving me to Shelton Hospital on the day of my discharge she warmed towards me. Later she became a good young psychiatric nurse and we got along fine. At least she was alright to my face and to me. I don't know how abusive she was when nobody was looking towards other patients.

Everybody has the potential to commit a crime and harm someone. In any given situation it can happen to anyone. People being frightened of you because you act strange is a completely different matter. But this is why most people end up being admitted to a psychiatric unit. Because of their strange behaviour, not because they have committed a crime or hurt anybody. You may say they have to be prevented from hurting themselves. But it is my argument that it is their right as owners of their own bodies and minds. Whether rational or otherwise. It is their right to do as they please with themselves. Saying that, I know I would go to the ends of the earth to save my son if he were in mortal danger from a suicide attempt. This is what every family member would do for their loved ones.

Anne E Watmough

Chapter 2 SUFFERAGE

Pankhurst Unit is named after Emeline Pankhurst who fought for the rights of women. She was born in Moss Side, Manchester, on the 15th July 1855 and died on 14th June 1928.

She lived in districts of Manchester I myself lived in, where I was raised. One district was Whalley Range next to Moss Side, and I lived there from the age of 13 until I married and after my brother died in 1977, when I was 24. So, she would have walked the same streets I walked.

She was born Emeline Goulden and married Richard Pankhurst when she was just 20 and he was 44. He was a barrister and they went on to have 5 children, one of which died in childhood, her only son at the time. She went on to have another son who she said was a reincarnation of the boy she lost.

For her convictions and beliefs Emeline was one of the first suffragists who spent time in jail. Her crimes were breaking windows, assaulting police officials and she was also accused of arson. She campaigned for votes for women.

It mustn't be forgotten just what she was up against. In fact, the whole of society and the then British establishment. Which still even today is largely ruled by men. What a brave lady to fight like she did. I am proud to have walked the same streets as she did.

I will never forget the first movement of suffragettes and what those women did in the name of justice for the likes of me. They went on hunger strike in prison. If anyone can imagine to be manhandled, roughed up and force fed with a tube placed into your mouth and down into your stomach, is a nice experience to have, then I suggest you need a psychiatrist more than I do.

Once asked if she would risk going to prison again in the future she said "Oh, yes quite. It wouldn't be so very dreadful you know, and it would be a valuable experience". One very brave and determined lady if ever there was one.

It wasn't just votes for women Emeline was fighting for. She was fighting against the conditions women and children found themselves in, in the workhouses and their living conditions.

In the workhouses of Manchester City children, girls of 8 and 9, were found scrubbing on their knees the stone floors along the long corridors there. Also, pregnant women who when there babies were born were in a very vulnerable position and they weren't safe. Don't forget this work was carried out in the heat of summer and the very cold of winter. I personally remember very cold winters during the I950's.

Emeline was a women of her time. She listened to the stories of women she lived with and who surrounded her daily life. Although she was an educated and middle class woman, having been sent to France for a lady's schooling, she had known her own hardship.

She had lost a child to diphtheria who was only little when he died. This left her grieving for some considerable time. She had known what it was like to be in need.

When she found herself taking care of her family including her parents and striving with her political work her and Richard believed she should not become a 'Household Machine'.

She fought for and brought about real change for the women of Britain. How many women of today would do the same for their fellow women? She befriended Kerr Harding the founder of the Labour Party. And had her rivals in the bad tempered and irritable Mainwairing a voice on the Board of Governors. She so irked him that he had to send constant notes to himself not to lose his temper. Probably Emeline was a thorn in his side.

What did Emeline Pankhurst do for me? If it wasn't for women like her who made it their business to be involved with politics and fight against the establishment, then not only would I not have the vote and my small say in the running of the country, I most probably would have found myself in a modern day version of the workhouse.

Emeline proved without a doubt that for the love of her grandmother, mother and daughters, a women's voice can be heard. And women can change their lives and the lives of others for the better.

Chapter 3 PRISON

Pankhurst Unit is a long vast corridor with rooms leading off on either side. There are utility rooms, bedrooms, doctor's interview rooms, waiting rooms, offices and rooms where some therapeutic practices are carried out. There is a coffee house where patients can go in another part of the hospital, but this isn't always open. There is also an isolation room. Every room is locked and unlocked by the staff.

I was given a room at the side of the dining area near to the kitchen and office. What I noticed almost immediately was the constant slamming of the kitchen and office doors. The doors were old and heavy and they slammed shut. I counted once that these doors were slammed shut by the nurses going in and out 60 times in 20 minutes. This wasn't during or just before or after mealtimes. And it was extremely noisy.

When you want a drink, or snack, you have to ask a nurse to get it for you. And you get served from a hatch through the kitchen door. So you are totally dependant on their goodwill. The same goes if you want to do your washing or for everything else. So, one thing you can guarantee, you are totally idle. You not only have time to think you have time to be bored off of your case. There is temporary occupational therapy which consists of making fruit smoothies, baking cakes, painting or playing bingo. When you make the smoothies you don't do that in a kitchen but in the O.T. Room. When you bake cakes you aren't always allowed in the kitchen which is off the ward. When painting they don't always have the paints and paper. The bingo has rubbish prizes. The food and meals are the highlight of your day is stodgy and puts weight on you along with the medication. So you end up with hardly any clothes that will fit you which you had brought in and they don't allow you to go shopping until much later in your stay and when they have the appropriate staff to accompany you. But there is still an awful lot of free time. The TV is in a perspex unit and under lock and key and you have to ask a member of staff for the remote. There is a WII and sometimes you can use this. But I never had the energy with what they were pumping into me. And tended to sleep my life away. The windows don't open and are sealed by a perspex cover. In the summer you can't open one window to let fresh air in and the air conditioning makes a horrendous noise when switched on.
Outside there are huge fences. In the courtyard there is a CCTV camera. There are no gardens and very little space to exercise.

There is a basket ball ring. Sometimes you find the energy to throw a ball.

I had a little radio that virtually kept me going. I had managed to acquire a battery charger just before I went into hospital and took that with me somehow when the social worker collected up some of my clothes for me. This charger was immediately placed into the office and plugged into a socket on the wall and I wasn't told until I spotted it and knew that it was mine. So I kept my eye on it as it might have taken the fancy of one of the staff. They are hard to come by apparently. There was a small safe in my room, so I managed to put all my important papers in there. This was a luxury I wasn't used to. But you couldn't keep the key to it yourself you had to ask for it and hand it back once you had got what you wanted from inside. So the staff could take a look at any private documents you had in your safe. ie solicitors letters etc.

I am not used to being in a hospital under lock and key and all my previous admittances have been in hospitals where I could go and come at my own pleasure. Because David Cameron is privatizing the National Health then these private hospitals have been set up for people like me to be detained. None of the other patients were violent either.

When somebody is emotionally traumatized and in need of sanctuary and peace so they can recuperate what they don't need is a noisy and hostile environment. They have not committed a crime against their fellow man/woman or themselves and they should not be punished. A peaceful environment with enough opportunity to reflect and understand one's circumstances and at the same time receive emotional assistance with empathy is not found in today's psychiatric hospital environments. And access to a curriculum of activities and things to occupy your time when you are capable to concentrate and not living in the haze of high toxic medication is desirable.

In fact another patient and I were watching a documentary on TV about life inside a prison and she pointed out to me that criminals receive more privileges than we do. They have access to see their children who are brought long distances and who can come and play in a nice colourful room. They have conjugal rights sometimes and can smoke in their cells and do not have to go outside in all weathers and be locked out. They receive education and are placed on work schemes and also they can earn some money by applying themselves to work projects within the prison. Not for people like me.

I have met in my time spent as an in-patient in psychiatric hospitals during the last 35 years some very good staff and patient's alike, but I have also met some awful ones too.

I have many memories, shock treatment has erased a few, but there are memories that are indelible on my mind and will remain with me until I die.

When I was a patient at The Priory I met the most wonderful women there. How they had survived for so long I will never know. Of course, without their permission, I cannot write much about them or mention their names. I can only briefly write about what I found.

I remember those women and one woman who became my friend. She was amazing. For many years she had been prescribed lithium and other toxic medications. Since the age of 16 she had been suffering from mania. When I met her she was in her 30's I would say, I don't know her age. These toxins were causing her to go blind and there would be no operation to save her sight.

Mainly suffering from mania she was hard to help by her family and also to nurse. People who suffer from mania sometimes think they are rich when in fact they have probably little finances. They run up debts of hundreds of pounds and their families usually have to bail them out. You can make bad financial decisions. I myself am prone to this also. But do not have a major problem with this.

There are other factors and the person can become so vulnerable and be in danger. So, family members also try and protect loved ones involved. Not because people in mania go about hurting others but they become a nuisance. My husband suffered from extreme mania and it used to be exhausting keeping up with him and trying to make sure he made no bad decisions and also that he was safe.

I ask this question, if a psychiatrist's diagnosis can be proved without a doubt that a person was in mania when buying or purchasing goods, then why is this person liable for the costs they incur? They have their liberty taken away from them and have no say in their treatment. So why are they liable for costs incurred when in a manic state? And why should family members find themselves in a position where they have to pay these debts back? It seems there are very few laws which protect these people and their families.

I also ask the question why should someone be forced or coerced into taking medication that is highly toxic and that the research proven that these drugs do what they actually say they do and cure the illness of madness has been done only by the drug companies themselves? When putting two and two together, it doesn't take a genius to think that this research could be in fact bogus especially as it is carried out in a laboratory on rats and mice. Then Macaw monkeys who might be our primate cousins but who are not human. Then on human guinea pigs. Which psychiatrists have access to. The research has been done that the long term use of psychotropic medications prolong symptoms of madness and give the very chemical imbalance bio psychiatrists say that you suffer from in the first place. Research is also being done by people like Professor David Healy that drug companies are corrupt and do not reveal their findings of drug research tests.

You could also question the integrity of nurses and doctors alike who allow somebody whilst in mania and difficult to nurse, because the nurses have not been trained with the correct procedures to care for this person, for a patient to be dragged by the hair down a long corridor and thrown into solitary. One to one nursing in this environment for somebody suffering from mania and confined to a small room with no chance of escape is torture. People in mania are over active and need space to roam and let off steam. They don't need to be brutally manhandled and confined in a small room for hours on end until they are sedated enough so that the running of the ward is easier for the nurses and patients alike. This happened to my friend and there has to be a better way.

The lady told me something about her past. How her parents had divorced when she was young and how her brother had sexually abused her. She had told nobody about this attempting to keep the family unit together and for fear she wouldn't be believed.

I remember how she would sing and dance and said she was from a showbiz family. It must have been in her blood. She would keep up moral with the other women. She had a fiance and they were planning a holiday for when she was discharged. Her mother visited her often and was devoted to her. Her friends would call her on her mobile. Along with her boyfriend who would constantly text her that he loved her very much. But this woman was strong willed and critical of her men folk, which years of abuse had brought about. She lived on her own a few blocks away from her mother. Who must have despaired at times and who probably brought her into the hospital wanting to protect her and not knowing the full consequences of what she had done. She had left my friend open and widely open to more abuse from men. Her psychiatrist being a man and the nurses with the most authority on the ward being male.

I remember how she became thirsty and had to drink a lot because of the lithium salts prescribed to her which she had been taking for years. If they did the job they were supposed to then why was she still being admitted to hospital? Years later? She, like others, did not deserve to be in a place which is not unlike a high security prison and where she was open to abuse. Simply because she was vulnerable and reaching a heightened state of reality and went into a manic state of mind.

There are eminent doctors out there, like Dr. Peter Breggin a formidable opponent to the corruption of drug companies and a reformist expert on psychiatric medications. He has won many a case in the American law courts for vulnerable people who have been damaged by these bio-psychiatrists and toxic drugs. Also he won with others victoriously the banishment of lobotomy throughout the West. Dr. Breggin is known as 'The Conscience of Psychiatry'. He has written numerous articles and published many books. Two novels also. My favourite of his books is 'The Psychology of Freedom' which was published the same year my son was born in 1980.

Other books are 'Toxic Psychiatry' and 'Brain Disabling Treatments in Psychiatry'. Amongst many books and articles he and his wife Ginger have a website and forum The Centre for the Study of Empathic Therapy, Education and Living which is also a new resource centre they have created in Syracuse, New York. He works as a regular psychiatrist in Ithaca, New York. To me I am dedicated to the man because he opened my eyes to just what was happening to me, which I was totally unaware of and assumed over and again was just me and my personal madness.

I believe strongly that there has to be a better way for people like my friend, myself and my son and so apparently does Dr. Breggin and his wife Ginger. There are others also. I hope that by writing my story change somehow will come about. However small that may be.

I spent a month in solitary at Shelton Hospital then one month on the Pankhurst Unit. And because I had accessed an advocate and was given a solicitor to contest my Section 3 and go to tribunal they had no choice but to let me go and discharge me.

The day of my discharge I was driven back from Stockport to Shrewsbury and just before I left I was again injected with something.

It was dark when my CPN came to take me home, the journey of 40 miles back to Wales. When we got through the front door into my house it was cold and damp and hadn't been occupied for two months. It was now the middle of January. I was so glad to return but there were memories of the fear I felt whilst in my paranoid state and I had to pick up the pieces yet again. I now live alone and my son was still in hospital.

Along the journey I talked to my CPN about Aliens. I felt during February 2010 I had had an encounter with an alien. Of course this was pure delusional. It was a wonderful delusion though and it was done simply by telepathy through the wall of my neighbours house who were all in bed at the time.

I simply loved this creature who had been on the Earth to assist and investigate us humans. His species had been of assistance to the authorities and the then prime minister of England and president of America which was George Bush.

He told me about the Nyx who were aliens with long limbs and who were blind but could sense people and animals by their sense of smell. They were dangerous only came out at night and made people disappear. He told me which planet he was from but I can't remember now. He was in charge of a fleet of space craft which were in the process of departing from earth and he was receiving messages and reports on how this was going. He said they had done all they could for us and he also said that this planet would be dead within 100 years. He said he would try and make room to evacuate my son if possible. And take him on board one of their space crafts which made long journeys in space.

He said that the Nyx capture people and before killing them they torture them and he asked me because I had had some military training would I work for George Bush? I said I couldn't do that and he told me what the Nyx did to people. So I said I would because I didn't want that happening to people or my son. He told me what planet he was from which I have forgotten now and that some of his kind were to remain here on the Earth to help out. This was my first delusion about aliens. But it was wonderful and now I do believe it possible for them to exist. It cannot be proven it is impossible.

Chapter 4 MADNESS

During February 2010 I did become quite insane. Because I came off all my medication abruptly. I asked my then psychiatrist if he would help me come off all my medication. Because I have been a revolving door patient for 35 years and they have never helped me. And he refused. And I began to withdraw after being on these drugs for 35 years. The withdrawal symptoms are the same as the illness itself. Paranoia, delusions and insomnia. In this state of mind and during the night at about 3am I went out to buy tobacco from my local all night garage in the town centre. It was pretty scary and I thought the Nyx were about but I had to prove my worth to this important and distinguished alien who wanted me for George Bush. I saw some people drive round a roundabout and I waved. Then I continued down the path and went into town and bought my tobacco. There was a car parked up so I thought I wonder if this person would give me a lift if I paid him £10 and I asked him and persuaded him to do this. In the back were two young teenagers giggling and both were young girls. I asked the driver if he was related to them and he said they had been to a party and he was taking them home for their mother. I asked the girls a couple of questions but didn't find out anything about them. Later I thought this really seemed suspicious. Because it was a school night.

I told my CPN that probably the first thing to go on earth would be transport. Because our resources are dwindling. It would be back to horses and carts and ships. I said I thought that aliens had arrived on earth generations ago and had always been around. But in the 1950's certain aliens had given us the knowledge of their technology. I said that I thought like Columbus when discovering islands in the pacific had given the natives of the islands gifts but also the common cold. And I thought that the aliens had given us technology which was like the common cold for humans today. Like a very contagious disease it was out of control.

Alan my then CPN said he thought maybe that going back to the basics and our roots might help humans to survive. But it will be an extremely hazardous journey because the Earth's climate is changing now. And the Earth's population has increased and that there would be 9 billion people living on earth in around thirty years times. I said I wondered if aliens were still around or if they had all left? Alan flinched.

When I got home I noticed bags of my belongings that I had in a state of panic been throwing out with the rubbish. I was so glad to find valuable sentimental items that I had kept for years and thought I had lost.

That night I forgot, probably because of the way the injection was affecting my train of thought, how to put my heating on. So I sat wrapped in a blanket shivering all night. After being home a few days I passed my neighbours house and saw their daughter cooking a roast dinner. I could smell it through their extractor fan and I was hungry. I looked in approvingly because she was cooking a roast during the week. This family's son had harassed and robbed me the year before in 2011.And was in prison at that time in January 2012 when I had just been discharged. I thought nothing about looking into their kitchen window. When I passed again they had put net curtains up and that morning when I went to go out there was a joint of beef on my front path. I thought the harassment had started again this time it was psychological.

My son left hospital three weeks later, but we still weren't discharged and are now on a Compulsory Treatment Order, which means we have to take the medication or else our psychiatrist can recall us back to hospital at any time if we refuse or miss an appointment with him, or the CPN. Once there in hospital they would force us against our will to take the medication. At higher doses.

For people like us who do not break the law or hurt people, why are we treated like criminals with even less rights than those who do commit crimes?

Some people, my late husband included, believe that medication has in fact cured them. But there is a large prognosis for what is known as the placebo affect. When somebody actually believes in something to such a depth and conviction then because human beings are so amazing we can actually cure ourselves of anything at all. I am not saying we are immortal, we all will die. I am not saying everything we suffer from is curable. But we can cure ourselves of most anything if we believe we can by either doing a certain ritual or believing something or someone will actually take away what ails us. Such is the capacity of the human mind, the brain, and the impact and control it has on our bodies and lives. I believe happiness is the key to curing madness and almost most of what ails us.

Our thinking is who we are. Our thoughts decide what we do with our lives and bodies. Nobody has the right to tell you what you should do with your own thoughts and your own body. They are yours and belong to nobody else.

And nobody can read your mind or tell you how to think. Nobody can control that. They can try, but the ultimate decision is your own. Deep inside everyone knows this. Even when a child we know this to be true.

As adults we like to control our children, mostly for their own good, but mostly because we can. Still children as small as they are know what is right and wrong to a certain extent and their thoughts are their own and you cannot enter into them.

Everybody has a right to their own inner sanctum and this always will be sacred. There should be no rules to say what you should feel and think, but psychiatrists feel they can and should do this to people who go mad. They coerce and force drugs on people. Most people who find themselves feeling and being in a heightened emotional crisis can be sorted by talking therapies and helped and never look back. Happiness can cure almost anything. The last World War and the Holocaust was particularly dangerous for mad people.

Before the power of the Nazis overtook Germany and its people they were experimenting on creating the super race. People who went mad and were disabled mentally or physically were sterilized. Then they were the first to be tortured and gassed . They were German, French and Polish people. Hitler and his henchmen wanted a super race and they wanted Germans to be that race and they desired to rule this race and therefore the world. Jews were prosperous, clever and shrewd. They created wealth. So they had to be rid of them all as they would get in their way. The way of creating the super race. Defects such as the mad were considered racially unhygienic. So they too had to be got rid of.

Some of the doctors who worked for the Nazis during the last World War went on to work in the psychiatric field after the War was over. In and around the 1950's chlorpromazine was discovered. Not as a cure for madness, but as a means of control. Because it subdued people and made them easier to either live with or to hospitalize.

You could say that mad people have had a raw deal throughout history. In the 16th century we were burnt at the stake, but never have so many been so cruelly damaged by the treatments of psychiatry over such a prolonged time then during the 20th century. Insulin induced comas and ice baths were used. With insulin comas a patient was injected with insulin which sent him into a coma then he was drastically brought out of it just as his life resources were closing down. With iced baths a patient was placed in a bath of iced water and strapped in then a cloth was placed over his eyes. He was kept there for several hours then once brought out he was wrapped in a recovery position with hot towels. One doctor used to drill into adult and children's brains through their eye sockets.

And today now at present nothing seems to have changed and it still continues. What is frightening and what some are aware of is that the so called "Mental Illnesses" seem to be affecting more and more people every day. It is my pure and unadulterated belief that there is no such thing as 'Mental Illness'. And I have suffered from madness since a little girl. The Mental Illnesses of today are simply describing how so many people are finding themselves unhappy. Also traumatized. We are told we should be happy and we should have all the worldly goods we desire. We should gamble on the lottery and win a fortune and that it is possible. We are entitled to a loving partner and loving happy children. If we find we cannot produce children we are taught we should be able and that this is our right too and is not impossible today. In other words we are told if we are unhappy with our lot in life we should strive for happiness. The danger lies in the fact that people are prescribed psychiatric medications and these are extremely harmful and can cause people to murder and even commit suicide. Especially the young.

We are taught that we should not accept even death the ultimate finality. If we don't have all we desire in this world we will be entitled to it in the next. But to me happiness is simply a state of mind. Doing or being forced to do something that makes us unhappy can lead to consequences sometimes which can become traumatic. Trauma can create dilemma and dilemma and the feeling of being trapped can cause the brain and mind to become mad.

I am not talking about people who suffer from dementia or alzheimers disease, these are diseases of the brain, but madness is not.

Families who find themselves in the responsible situation of care for a loved one who suffers with their insanity have very little support and have no alternative but to admit this family member to hospital and because of the lack of education about madness and all other emotional crisis then they too become overwhelmed in some respects.

This and the stigma and time consuming tasks in taking care of an individual who becomes incapacitated and acting strange and not themselves can be so distressing for families and family members. If a family member commits suicide this can be devastating on every family member and can affect people like no other death can. Their only help are social services, GP's, psychologists and psychiatrists. Who in the UK are bio-psychiatrists. In the past the stigma of madness was so acute in society that even aristocrats who unfortunately gave birth to handicapped children had to have them institutionalized. The diagnoses then given by doctors was 'Imbecile'. It is to my own knowledge and experience that many mentally handicapped mentally challenged people are very loving and also very talented and can be despite their disabilities extremely knowledgeable and intelligent.

For families of people living during the Victorian era and even to the present day the stigma of madness is so embedded in our society that although people want to devote themselves to there own flesh and blood that choice is taken away from them. And people find themselves many times having to abandon their relatives and give them over to institutions and these doctors.

Like someone recently said to me treating trauma with trauma is not the right way to help people like myself who live with losing their mind. Fear is no stranger to me. When fear attacks my thoughts I live with it 24/7 for maybe days on end. When you are sent to a place of jeopardy then this becomes a no win vicious lifestyle. The "Double Bind". Dr. R. D. Laing wrote in his book whereby a person can find herself in a situation where to make one decision would be detrimental and to make another would bring her into a harmful situation. A person can find themselves in a situation where there is only two decisions which have to be made and each of these decisions is detrimental to that person.

Personally when I am mad I feel that my psychiatrist is liken to that of a Black Widow Spider. He being the female and me being the male and I am in the precarious position of being eaten at any time. Trapped in his web I am wrapped in silk and every time I struggle to become free the more entangled I become. My only hope for freedom and escape is to maybe bite through the threads and for the sweet embrace of many rain drops to wash me away down into the undergrowth below and to safety. To a place where I can find my freedom and ultimately my peace.

Anne E Watmough

22

Chapter 5 MAD AND HILARIOUS

Whilst at Shelton on Stokesay Ward I formed a relationship with a lady who seemed quite rational most of the time. She became my ally and was the only one to tell me Lee had a broken arm, until locked away on High Dependency, she didn't notice my little face trying to gain her attention through the tiny window on the door.

The last time we met was on the day I returned for my discharge. Whilst this lady and I went outside so she could draw on her rolly because the rules are patient's have to evacuate themselves outside for a smoke. And there are pleasantly situated pergolas placed outside each ward where patient's are obliged to sit and enjoy their Condor moments.

There are four open sides to these little smoking retreats, so when the weather is bad you are exposed to the elements and it is somewhat like trying to enjoy a fag whilst enduring a snow blizzard in the Arctic if it is raining and windy.

Alas, night time becomes a problem if you desire to smoke when for security reasons everything is locked and only staff can go in and out. Saying that, most of the time these exits are locked during the day also and so many times I have seen people knocking on the glass door to be let in. Outside in all weathers wondering why on earth they just couldn't simply kick the habit. But with nothing at all else to do with one's endless eternal time and when boredom seeps in amongst unreality and the gagging of emotional expression, then smoking seems quite an innocent crime.

The woman I mentioned and I went out on this particular sunny winter's day and sat on a bench. I had quit the habit a few years earlier. She told me how she had been sending off letters to the Health Authority requesting to be placed on a Section 3 not a Section 6 of the Mental Health Act and had made numerous phone calls, but as yet to no avail. Me being bent on escape didn't quite grasp what it was she was telling me. I didn't realize the lower the number the higher the section.

She told me a little about herself. That she lived in a big rambling house where she had grown up. That her mother had passed away some time back and there was just her and her brother left.

Before parting I said to her I hoped she would be leaving soon and not have to wait long before going home. Her exact words were 'No, I don't want to leave. I want to stay here forever. I want a higher Section'. Then I just fell about laughing and we must have belly laughed for ten minutes.

They say laughter is the best medicine. It certainly can help any emotional crisis. My husband had the most witty and dry sense of humour. Pity psychiatrists don't see the joke?

She gave me a wonderful book of poems by John Clare. I wondered afterwards just what her brother must have been like to live with? And did he ever go crazy?

Chapter 6 LOVE

It is a sunny warm Spring day with clear blue skies and I have just returned from Blackpool. I went there to see my mum who was staying in a guest house with my aunty. I was hoping to stay there with them only aunty wouldn't pay for me.

I had called my psychiatrist and asked if I could be admitted onto ward P10 and he agreed.

So, there I was three weeks from my 26th birthday being admitted into Withington Psychiatric Hospital in the city of Manchester where I grew up. This had been about my second admission so far.

I sat myself down with my little battered red suitcase by my side and a dark handsome tanned young man approached me and started to talk.

Mancunians like many northerners are very open, so it wasn't long before Mark got the low-down on me and found out what had led me to be there on that warm Spring day in May l977.

I had just ended an affair that went badly and my brother had hung himself a few weeks earlier. I couldn't bare staying in the bedroom next to his where he did it, what with my mum away and only my dad in the house for company, who I felt took some part in it. My dad during a phone call with me years later told me that on the night David took his life he told my dad and dad said to my brother not to talk about it but to go ahead and do it. I knew at the time dad had something to do with it. But I forgive him and realize it was a desperate situation.

I had to get away somehow.

On that day on Ward P10 when I met Mark for the first time before he went back to his ward the admittance ward P1, he wrote his name, address and telephone number on a little white card and I kept it for 33 years. Then just recently I lost it. I wasn't to know he would become my future husband, the father of my only child and the love of my life.

I latched onto my friend Andrew who I knew from before. Andrew's father was the top consultant at Christies Cancer Hospital and ironically his own mother had breast cancer and had to have a mastectomy.

Andrew was a diagnosed schizophrenic like me. When he was not overcome by his madness he was part of the 70's jet set and knew people like the model in the Cadbury's Chocolate Flake advert. Andrew was gay, and I was in awe of him. At around my early 20's I too had been part of the then so called jet-set and hung around with the Georgie Best crowd. Georgie Best was the first glamorous celebrity footballer and played for Manchester United in the 1970s.

My friend Eva and I used to go to the clubs Blinkers and Samantha's. And once we were invited to an Xmas party at Georgie Best's house. There was an Xmas tree in one part of the room and underneath were hundreds of cards from his fans. The famous entertainer Kenny Lynch was there at that time.

One night whilst I was dancing at Samantha's Georgie approached me wanting to dance with me and I am afraid I turned my back on him. The reason being a few nights earlier a stunning blonde bombshell came into the ladies loo and told us that Georgie had taken her back to his house the night before. Because she wouldn't have sex with him he threw her out and she had to walk home in the dark in the early hours by herself. This was long before mobile phones were invented.

It wasn't that George wasn't handsome, he was incredibly so, but under the influence of drink a lovely natured young man became a monster. For him to gain the right help he needed all of his childhood experiences and a lifetime of emotional crisis to be addressed, understood challenged and he needed to be given the emotional tools in which to cope with this but like I have witnessed so many times, people are given anti-abuse, told to refrain from the demon drink and go cold turkey. Whatever had caused Georgie Best to drink never went away and left him and eventually it was his downfall. For such an incredible athlete and nice natured person this to me was a sad tragedy that his life was blighted so.

Once when I was sat at the bar in Blinkers Jimmy Tarbuck the famous comedian of the 60's and 70's approached me and commented that I had nice boobs. I wasn't showing a cleavage and basically was covered, and this wasn't a come-on, it was a compliment and I took it as such. He went back to his wife and friends who were sat at a table and their laughter rang out of the club on that night.

Around this time I applied to the Sheila Wilson model agency to become a model. They were looking for skinny skinny and she told me I was very pretty but not what they were looking for. I did get accepted by the Lucy Clayton agency though and ended up doing some escort work with a very lovely girlfriend who was a Mormon. We met these two Italian men who were over from Naples on holiday here. I ended up having sex with Giovani who was quite gorgeous and we met up again when I went over to work in Italy. He took me out along the Amalfi coast which was so beautiful also he invited me and my friend Lyn for a meal at his house with his family.

Before I went to work in Italy I applied at the Playboy Club to become a Bunny Girl. They gave me a job to train on the roulette tables but I wasn't confident about doing the maths so I didn't go.

Back then as a 22 year old I knew nothing about psychiatry. I had read a few good books and one on Gestalt Therapy, but I was under the impression that psychiatrists were knowledgeable, trained and experienced. I didn't realise that their silence was in fact because they had no idea at all how to deal with your emotional crisis and problems. All that bio-psychiatrists know and believe in is medication and finding the drug that suits you. The damage it does to your moods and therefore your feelings is overlooked and they class as your illness.

Almost 40 years later I know the truth and the full facts, but I am also aware that the general public do not know at all. And people don't know the affects of psychiatric drugs on their minds and bodies.

Chapter 7 THE WELSH POET

In 1951 Dylan Thomas wrote about the Great Exhibition held in London:

The extent of the site of the exhibition on the South Bank of the Thames in the heart of London is four and a half acres. There are twenty-two pavilions in the exhibition, and thirteen restaurants, cafes, bars and buffets.

Some people visit the twenty-two pavilions first, then glazed and crippled, windless, rudderless, and a little out of their minds, teeter, weeping, to one of the thirteen restaurants, cafes, bars, and buffets to find it packed to the dazzlingly painted and, possibly,levitating doors.

Other people visit all thirteen restaurants, cafes, bars, and buffets before attacking the pavilions, and rarely get further than the Dome of Discovery, which they find confusing, full, as it is, of totem poles, real dogs in snow, locusts, stars, the sun, the moon, things bubbling, thunder and lightning machines, chemical and physical surprises. And some never return.

Most people who wish, at the beginning, anyway, to make sense of the exhibition, follow the course indicated in the official guidebook – a series of conflicting arrows which lead many visitors who cannot understand these things slap-splash into the Thames – and work their way dutifully right through the land of Britain, the glaciers of twenty thousand years ago, and the inferno of blown desert sand which is now Birmingham, out at last into the Pavilion of Health – where, perhaps, they stop for an envious moment at the sign that says 'Euthanasia' - and on the netted and capstaned, bollarded, buoyed, sea-shelled pebbly beautiful seaside of summer childhood gone.

And other visitors begin, of course, at the end. They are the people without whom the exhibition could not exist, not the country it trombones and floats in with its lions and unicorns made of ears of wheat, its birds that sing to the push of a button, its flaming water, and its raspberry fountains. They are the suspicious people over whose eyes no coloured Festival wool can possibly be pulled, the great undiddleable; they are the women who 'will not queue on any account' and who smuggle in dyspeptic dogs; the strangely calculating men who think that the last pavilion must be first because it is number twenty-two; the people who believe they are somewhere else, and never find out they are not; sharp people who have been there before who know the ropes, who chuckle to their country cousins: 'You get double your money's worth this way'; vaguely persecuted people, always losing their gloves, who know that the only way they could ever get around would be to begin at the end, which they do not want to; people of militant individuality who proclaim their right, as Englishmen, to look at the damfool place however they willynilly will; people nervously affected by all such occasions, who want to know only, 'Where's the place?'; timid people who want to be as far from the skylon as possible, because 'you never know'; foreigners, who have been directed this way by a school of irresponsible wits; glassy benighted men who are trying to remember they must see something of the exhibition to remember before they go home and try to describe it to their families; young people, hand-in-love, who will giggle at whatever they see, at a goldfish in a pond, a model of the Queen Elizabeth, or a flint hammer; people too bored to yawn, long and rich as borzois, who before they have seen it, have seen better shows in Copenhagen and San Francisco; eccentric people: men with their deerstalker caps tied with rope to their lapels, who carry dried nut sandwiches and little containers of yoghurt in hairy green knapsacks labelled 'glass with care'; fat, flustered women in as many layers of coats as an onion or a cab-driver, hunting in a fever through fifty fluffed pockets to find a lost packet of bird-seed they are going to give to the parrots who are not there; old scaly sneezing men, born of lizards in a snuff-bin, who read, wherever they go, from books in tiny print, and who never look up, even at the tureen-lid of the just-tethered dome or the shining skylon, the skygoing nylon, the cylindrical leg-of-the-future jetting, almost, to the exhibition of stars; real eccentrics; people who have come to the South Bank to study the growth and development of Britain from the Iron Age till now. Here they will find no braying pageantry, no taxidermal museum of Culture, no cold and echoing inhuman hygienic barracks of technical information,no shoddily cajoling emporium of tasteless Empire wares, but something very odd indeed, magical and parochial: a parish-pump made of flying glass and thistledown gauze-thin steel, a rolypoly pudding full of luminous, melodious bells, wheels, coils, engines and organs, alembics and jorums in a palace in thunderland sizzling with scientific witches' brews, a place of trains, bones, planes, ships, sheep, shapes, snipe, mobiles, marbles, brass bands, and cheese, a place painted regardless, and by hand.

Perhaps you'll think I'm shovelling the colour on too thickly; that I am, as it were, speaking under the influence of strong pink, (And what a lot of pink- rose, raspberry, strawberry, peach, flesh, blush, lobster, salmon, tally-ho – there is, plastered and doodled all over the four-acre gay and soon-to-be-gone Festival City in sprawling London.) London: to many of us who live in the country, the Capital punishment. Perhaps you will go on a cool, dull day, sane as a biscuit, and find that the exhibition does, indeed, tell the story 'of British contributions to world civilization in the arts of peace'; that, and nothing else. But I'm pleased to doubt it. Of course it is instructive; of course there is behind it an articulate and comprehensive plan, it can show you, unless you are an expert, more about, say, mineralogy or the ionosphere than you may want to know. It's bursting its buttons, in an orderly manner, with knowledge. But what everyone I know, and have observed, seems to like most in it is the gay, absurd, irrelevant, delighting imagination that flies and booms and spurts and trickles out of the whole bright boiling; the small stone oddity that squints at you round a sharp, daubed corner; the sexless abstract sculptures serenely and secretly existing out of time in old cold worlds of their own in places that appear, but only for one struck second, in appropriate; the linked terra-cotta man and woman fly-defying gravity and elegantly hurrying up a W.C. Wall; the sudden design of hands on another wall, as though the painter had said: 'Oh, to the daft devil with what I'm doing.' and just slap-slap-slapped all over the ochre his spread-out fingers and thumbs, ten blung arrows, or as though large convict-birds, if there are any such, had waddled up the wall and webbed it as they went. You see people go along briskly down the wide white avenues towards the pavilion of their fancy – 'Our Humbert's dead keen on seeing the milk-separators'- and suddenly stop: another fancy swings or bubbles in front of their eyes. What is it they see? Indigo water waltzing to music. Row after row of rosy rolling balls spread on tall screens like the counting beads of Wellsian children fed on the food of the gods. Sheets of asbestos tied on to nowhere, by nothing, for nothing is anchored here and at the clap of hands the whole gallimaufry could take off to Sousa and zoom up the flagged sky. Small childbook-painted mobiles along the bridges that, at a flick of wind, become windmills and thrum round at night like rainbows with arms. Or the steel-and-platinum figure – created by the Welsh engineer and architect, Richard Huws – of maybe a mer-woman standing, if that is the word for one who grows out of it, in arc-light water; she weeps as she is wept on; first her glinting breast, then another plane of her, tips, slides, shoots, shelves, swings and sidles out to take, from the late of her birth, one tone of water at a time to Handel's Water Music, absorbs it, inhales it through dripping steel, then casts and cascades it off and out again. Or even the hundreds of little vivid steel chairs that look like hundreds of little vivid steel people sitting down.

In the pavilion called 'The Natural Scene', see the seals and eagles, the foxes and wild cats, O these still wild islands, and the natural history of owled and cuckooed, ottered, unlikely London. A

31

great naked tree climbs on the middle of all, with prodigious butterflies and beetles on it. A blackbird lights up, and the aviary's full of his singing; a thrush, a curlew, a skylark.

And, in the 'Country', see all the sculpted and woven loaves, in the shape of sheaves of wheat, in curls, plaits, and whirls. And men are thatching the roofs of cottages; and – what a pleasure of baskets! Trugs, creels, pottles and punnets, heppers, dorsers and mounds, wiskets and whiskets. And if these are not the proper words, they should be.

In 'The Lion and the Unicorn' is celebrated, under flights O birds, the 'British Character', that stubborn, stupid seabound, lyrical, paradoxical dark farrago of uppishness, derring-do, and midsummer moonshine of fluting, snug, and copper-bottomed. Justice, for some reason, looms in the midst of the Hall, its two big wigs back to back. Its black and scarlet robes falling below. The body of justice is shelves of law books. The black spaces beneath the white wigs looks like the profiles of eagles. The white knight rides there too, too much a Don Quixote for my looking-glass land, and very potless and panless. A bravo-ing hand pats his plaster back, and tells him good night. There is a machine for, I believe, grinding smoke. And a tea-set, I failed to see, of salmon bones. But, in all this authentically eccentric exhibition, it is the Eccentrics' Corner that is the most insipid. Some of the dullest exhibits in the pavilion are relieved by surrounding extravagance; but the department devoted to the rhapsodic inspirations of extravagance is by far the dullest. Why was not the exquisite talent utilized of the warlock who, offering his services to the Festival authorities, assured them he would, to order, throw a rainbow over the Thames? I wish he would throw a rainbow over me as I walk through the grey days. 'Yes, we can tell it's him coming,' the envious neighbours would murmur, 'we recognize his rainbow.' And, on the balcony, there is a row of tiny theatres; in each, the stage is set for a Shakespearian play, and out of the theatres come the words of the players. If you're in luck, something may go wrong with the works and Hamlet rant from Dunsinane.

In 'Homes and Gardens', blink at the grievous furniture, ugly as sin and less comfy.

In the 'Transport Pavilions', goggle at the wizard diesels and the smashing, unpuffing streamlines and the miracle model railway for dwarf nabobs.

Then, if there are by this time no spots in front of your eyes, go to the Tlecinema and see them astonishingly all around you: spots with scarlet tadpole tails, and spottedly sinuous tintacks dancing with dissolving zebra heads, and blobs and nubbins and rubbery squirls receding, to zig-zag blasts of brass, down nasty polychrome corridors, a St Virus's gala of abstract shapes and shades in a St Swithin's day of torrential dazzling darning needles. Sit still in the startling cinema and be kissed by a giraffe, who stretches his neck right out of the screen for you. Follow the deliberately coloured course of the Thames, the Royal River; the whispering water's more like water than water ever was; closer, closer, comes the slow kingfisher – blue water and suddenly it ripples all over you: that'll be the day when film stars do the same.

Go to the South Bank first by day; the rest of your times at night. Sit at a cafe table in the night of musical lights, by the radiant river, the glittering skylon above you rearing to be off, the lit pavilion , white, black, and silver in sweeps of stone and feathery steel, transplendent round you as you sip and think:

This is the first time I have ever truly seen that London whose sweet Thames runs softly; that minstrel mermaid of a town, the water-streeted eight -million-headed village in a blaze. This is London, not the huge petty misshaped nightmare I used to know as I humdrummed along its graceless streets through fog and smoke and past the anonymous unhappy bodies lively as wet brollies. This Festival is London. The arches of the bridges leap into light; the moon clocks glow, the river sings; the harmonious pavilions are happy. And this is what London should always be like, till St. Paul's falls down and the sea slides over the Strand.

This is what Dylan Thomas wrote in a broadcast during 1951 about the Festival Exhibition.

Chapter 8 BEGINNINGS

I was born Anne Elizabeth Lozinski on the 16th June 1951. My birth took place in St. Mary's Hospital, Prestbury, Macclesfield in Cheshire. The only one of us to be born in hospital being mum's first. From what mum told me it was a normal birth and she remembered whilst being examined by the doctor he slapped her on the bottom. She said how embarrassing this was at the time and this doctor was handsome. She was tanned and healthy and wore her shining black hair tied back on her shoulders in a snood.

A year later my eldest brother came along, then three years later my younger brother then five years later my baby sister. I remember her being born when I was five years old and the midwife asked me to bring a bowl of warm water to help mum. I will never forget the sweet smell of birth and how much I loved having such a delightful baby and child to take care of.

My earliest memory was when I was a baby and I recall how I loved my mother's smell. It was probably the smell of mother's milk the life giving force needed by infants. I attached myself to that and the bond between mother and baby was strong. I too breast fed my son for six months, until I was hospitalized and drugged when it was no longer possible.

Whilst I was carrying my son I was drug and medication free. I didn't smoke. I was healthy and rode my bicycle everywhere. The air was fresh and my diet was good. I was happy and so was Mark.

I know of mothers who whilst carrying their child are prescribed psychiatric medications. This is barbaric along with the treatment of so called ADHD for normal healthy children with emotional problems. Babies are born deformed and children are damaged with Ritalin on their young growing brains for the rest of their natural lives. This has to stop. Legislation has to come about to stop this barbaric treatment of a mother in distress whilst pregnant with her child.

A baby's early attachment to it's mother Carl Gustav Jung describes as the 'cupboard love' theory. Reading Jung and Freud is not boring or difficult to me and I am particularly interested in the women who were involved with them. Fraud based all his psychotherapy conclusions on his theories about sexuality and the suppressed feelings stemming from childhood. Fraud's theories were based on what he described as the Oedipus Complex which is when a young male child reaches the age of say 4 or 5 years and becomes aware that like his father he has a penis and that his mother and sisters don't have one. Freud concluded that a young boy falls in love with his mother and thinks that his sisters have been castrated. Therefore he becomes threatened by his father's part in his relationship with his mother and becomes envious and this affects the relationship with his mother therefore if it is a difficult one the Oedipus Complex is contrived and this leads to neurosis and psychological difficulties later in life. Also it is my belief that this can create homosexuality in men. But the theory totally cannot be applied to females and the female child and Freud did not have a verifiable conclusion about this and the affect of a mother-daughter relationship on personality and therefore what creates neurosis and madness in women later in life. Freud based his conclusions about little girls wanting their fathers to penetrate them and to be seduced and therefore feeling inferior because they don't have a penis. This is of course farcical.

But as far as psychotherapy goes there seems to be a popular craze for CBT which basically attempts to change your whole way of thinking. I do not want my way of thinking changed I might benefit from looking at things in a different perspective but I don't want my way of thinking messed with.

I think to overlook the study and mystery of dreams is dangerous if we must explore the integrities of our brains and minds. We only use a small part of our brains as far as we have evolved at this present day and age.

For these past three years I have consulted an existential psychotherapist I discovered on the Mind Freedom website. He is a qualified in the existentialist psychotherapy. Which means his basis for treatment if formed on the foundations of Existentialism. Simone de Beauvoir is a famous French feminist writer who lived in France and was born in Paris in 1908. She was a very educated and prolific writer. The love of her life was Sartre. Together they based their beliefs on this philosophy. Her most famous book is titled The Second Sex.

Existentialism is of the belief that an individual is a free agent who is burdened with personal responsibility. And whose existence cannot be investigated objectively. Being revealed by reflection on existence in time and space. It tends to dispel scientific methodology and knowledge and to reject objective values.

This therapist my first ever happened to be the right one for me. There are different types of therapy and sometimes changing therapists to find one that suits you is imperative if you feel you are getting nowhere. But Mick has been so wonderfully helpful to me. He has understood where I was coming from been non judgemental and been there by text which he gives free along with his emails every day.

My therapy with Mick Bramham has been life changing. For the first time in my life I could actually talk about myself and my madness to a person I knew would not judge and who was not involved with me emotionally. Would advise and reassure objectively and with affection.

I owe Mick so very much. And will always be in his debt. I now know that I am cured of my madness and will continue as long as possible to consult him about the issues in my life. He is quite a remarkable person. Having a history of working with young disturbed boys in a residential home whose head did not believe in medication. And then going on to work in a charity raising over £1,000,000 in funds for the good of people with emotional difficulties. Like being homeless etc.

Mick lives in a 17th century cottage in Dorset and was plagued by a flood. He has spent the last few years restoring his home. He adores and loves dogs. Anyone who adores and loves dogs has my utmost respect.

He has met some of the most wonderful people I most admire and believes like me society has such a large play in our lives. Society is like the body made up of tiny cells. We are those tiny cells. Each cell profoundly as important as the next to keep the body alive and living. When cells die part of the body dies. Mick's website is Risks & Myths.

Carl Jung wrote about the Collective Unconsciousness. I believe this exists. This is what we call the media today. How we are all tuned in to the areas we live in and what is going on with people around us. Basically our culture.

I believe like my father in telepathy. I believe everybody's thoughts go out into the world and are connected. I don't believe you can read someone's mind. I believe like my husband that we each have a telepathic partner and can connect with this person freely.

My husband had telepathy. He could find me no matter where I was. I know I had telepathy with my cat Whiskas. When I first met Mark he had a friend who was engaged to a German industrialist. Mark said he would help her and believed they were telepathic partners. He said any time she needed him to think of her favourite soft toy Twinkle. To think of the word "Twinkle" and he would be there for her. So one day he was up on P10 with me and said suddenly he had to go and that Sarah needed him. And when he went down to see her he asked if she was alright and she said she was she just lost her temper for a few minutes and threw her soft toy Twinkle down on the floor.

One of my earliest memories are of my Uncle Kazik, my dad's brother. I remember a warm loving kind funny man who took me with him everywhere and bought me dresses and shoes and toys. There was a time I recall walking down the street with Kazik and asking him if when I grew up could we get married. Where was the logic of this in the mind of a child?

I vaguely still remember what he looked like and there are photographs of us together taken at a studio.

Kazik was the only one in the whole family to be physically injured during the last World War. He was driving a truck in a convoy of the Red Cross when hit by enemy fire and badly injured. His companion carried him on his back for 8 miles to the nearest hospital and Kazik's life was saved. He had a scar down one side of his handsome face.

My mother told me years later why Kazik left suddenly and was never to return. That he confronted dad about his domestic violence and the quarrels mum and dad were having at the time. Dad accused him of interfering and they argued and dad threw Kazik out into the street. Kazik then left England, went back to Poland and never returned. He married a Polish lady and had six children of his own.

When on my wedding day to Mark he sent me a tape on which he wished me every happiness I remembered his kindness and warmth and the love I felt for this uncle. When he left so abruptly I was little and under those circumstances it must have been one of my first childhood experiences of trauma. I must have missed him terribly and this will always lye in my subconscious even though the memory is lost to me the feeling of loss will never be forgotten.

When I was three years old one day during the Summer I was sunning myself on a garden wall when I got the bright idea that I had to experience just what it was like to actually fall off. Mum must have warned me to be careful. So I did just that, I leant forward and fell off down onto the pavement below. I had the most massive swollen forehead and had to be taken by ambulance to the Infirmary. I could have had concussion and had to be X-rayed. I have had a small lump on my forehead for the rest of my life. It seemed I had to experience everything then and continued to think that way all of my life. I was a tomboy as a girl and a romantic and feminist in adult life.

My mother used to sit us around the open coal fire and sing to us from songs she made up out of her imagination. She used to tell us stories too not from written books but from her own thoughts and imagination. Every Friday when possible and dad was in work she would give us pocket money and send us to the local shop for toffees and chocolates. Also bottles of cream soda, orange juice and dandelion and burdock. She would simply ask us to buy one block of Caramac chocolate or whole nut bar of chocolate for herself. Then when we had eaten all of ours she would share hers with us. Her pleasures were little in her life. One thing she did enjoy were her books and she was an avid reader. When we were somewhat older and she had the time she would read about 2 to 3 books in a week and then short stories and belonged to two large libraries in the city.

Dad would constantly bring home musical instruments like accordions or trumpets. We had a piano in our front parlour. But because dad had never learnt how to play properly and his schooling had been interrupted so brutally when he was a young man of 18 and attending college then we never learnt to play and he could never afford lessons for us. It must have been a huge disappointment that all his efforts were in vain. But, my brother when grown taught himself to play guitar and his children are very artistic and musically talented. My son also is artistically talented. My brother is an artist and I too can sketch and paint. I felt my husband had his own unique artistic talent also. And Lee is good at painting and drawing. He can play guitar and the drums also a little.

At around the same time my sister was born I attended primary school for the first time. I went to St. Joseph's Catholic School. I wanted to continue playing in the sandpit and the teacher thought otherwise so I kicked her in the shins and ran home to mum. I was subsequently marched back military style the next morning and learnt my first important lesson in life. Just where I stood in the scheme of things. A harsh but oh so valuable lesson.

My next teacher when I must have been 6 years old was bent on teaching us all how to sing. She taught us to open our mouths wide and let our voices flow out loud and strong. To pronounce our diction and pronunciation and let our singing ring out. Unfortunately, not everyone has a voice worth listening to and in tune and I am afraid I am tone deaf. But I enjoyed her class.

The best teacher we had in primary school was Mrs. Brennan. She was married with a family of her own and knew something about children. Because my home life was in crisis and my parents were struggling financially my school work did suffer. Also we were as children exposed to the abuse of domestic violence between our parents. Constant rowing and fighting had been the norm between them especially in the early years of their marriage.

I started to copy my friend's work and passed the class test with flying colours. But then I was sent to a higher class and of course couldn't do the work so became second to bottom. Mrs Newton mainly taught maths. Ralph who sat next to me was bottom. No point in copying his work. We were both two first class dunces. I used to find it traumatic having to stand at the front of the class by the teacher's side at her desk and try and work out sums. I could not get the hang of it. Not that I wasn't bright it was the whole way I was being taught. As a ten year old with no knowledge whatsoever of the subject. And the constant fear of being laughed at and made fun of by my peers.

Whilst online once I discovered a new education centre of excellence which had been built in America. I listened to a talk given by one of its founders who was a mathematician. He explained how every child has the capacity to learn and master maths. That he and his colleagues were introducing new methods of teaching that were revolutionizing the way in which young children as early as three could be introduced and taught how to master maths and mathematical problems. That there was no need for any child not to achieve this education. This new teaching approach was to be introduced to state primary schools in America.

But many children feel inferior when they don't achieve top marks at school and most decide not to devote their energies on lessons. They get disillusioned and decide to drop out and concentrate on fashion, pop music and popular trends. Smoking and drinking and things to blot out and find some sort of fun in their struggling lives. Saying that there are so many youngsters who work hard and are conscientious with school work and who also find themselves unable to get good positions of employment once leaving school or college. Quite a few young people succeed and excel and go on to prosper even in today's climate of austerity.

I had a friend who had a Nigerian father and Scottish mother. She was poor. But highly intelligent. She was the only black girl in my school. Philomeana was the first person to tell me she thought I had an inferiority complex. At ten years old her clever but struggling mother had known I suffered from this. Phil's dad had left them and I lost touch when we left Chorlton- on- Medlock and went to live in Victoria Park. One night I walked in the pouring rain to see her and as always she wouldn't let me come into her home. They were so poor and her sister wouldn't allow anyone inside. I often think of her and our times together when we were both ten years old.

I remember walking home from school with Phil and once a woman called us into her house along Mornington Street to see her little girl who had just died of leukaemia. She was like a large beautiful doll placed in an upright box. Laid out in a silk embroidered lace dress with tiny pretty white shoes and surrounded in satin ruffles. Her hair was blonde and in ringlets. Her pretty little face with eyes which had long dark lashes was covered in little spots but nevertheless this child was so loved and even in death she was adored by a mother who wanted to display her to the world. Before finally laying her in the ground and losing sight of her forever.

Our last class before leaving primary school was in Mr. Willoughby's. He was a monster and abused the 11 year olds under his care. I remember he picked on one boy in particular constantly berating and humiliating him in front of the class. One day he beat him down one aisle of the class and up the other. I just kept my head down and tried to avoid him.

Five years later when my sister was also in his class she was having a reading period when she finished her book. Wanting to be a good pupil she approached Mr. Willoughby at his desk and asked if she could replace her book from the bookshelf for a new one to read. She thought this was what he wanted her to do. Then for no reason he struck her across the face so hard her nose bled and wouldn't stop. She had to be taken to the Royal Infirmary and my mother went up to the class and told him just what she would do to him if he ever did anything like that again.

His excuse! 'She wasn't to interrupt him when he was marking books!' A man with major problems. This was a particularly disgusting act as Janet is only petite and was a tiny child. Janet said this monster of a teacher went on to be the headmaster of St. Joseph's Primary School. Later my sister told me she had found out he had died in a fire. But before that he had been promoted to Headmaster of the school.

Violence it appeared had become the norm for us in our childhood years, but we all became good adults and no crime committers. Among all of this turmoil there was in fact happiness and we must have been given an awful amount of love and affection to turn into the adults we did eventually become. There were many times of solace happiness and adventure.

My dad is Polish and when he was in college at the age of 18 Germany sold out on Poland. First of all Germany invaded Poland in 1944 which made the then British prime minister Neville Chamberlain declare war on Germany against Hitler.

Then there was a pact with Poland and Russia where Russia proclaimed to become allies with Poland. They entered the country as allies and in fact it was an invasion. My father remembers Russians on horse back riding through the street with swords hacking people down who were running for their lives. He also was running for his life and along with his brother hid in a shop doorway and escaped death by sword.

At the age of 18 he was attending college and a Russian speaker was in class before this happened. Dad became suspicious and the next thing he knew he was being interrogated. Then the Russians showed their true colours and started to round people up and he was sent to a concentration camp in Siberia.

They ransacked Poland on horseback hacking people down with swords. A horseman was just about to strike my father who had been hiding in a doorway with his younger brother Marion when mistaken in his school uniform for a soldier. A woman cried out "No he is a youngster spare him!"

In order to qualify for food in the camp men had to fell trees and dad being only slight in stature found this really difficult and couldn't do it. A man has to be quite strong to fell a tree. So he was starving and he thought how on earth can I survive this? He got the idea to play for his supper and formed a small band because he could play the violin and someone else the accordion another the trumpet and they entertained the people which qualified him to receive food and this kept him alive.

After my dad was in the camp when the liberating Americans and British were approaching and the Russian army were dying because of the harsh winter in Siberia he was released. Travelling across Europe along with other refugees he settled in one place to sleep and was quite cold. He was under a bunk when lice started to fall on him and the person above who had been wearing a fur coat had died so they were all jumping ship and ended up falling on my dad.

He never returned to Poland until after my mother passed away in 1997. In 1985 my 91 year old grandmother came over to England to see us all. She had never flown before in her life. What a remarkable woman. She could not speak English and I no Polish but we sat next to each other holding hands. There were tears in her eyes when she said goodbye to us all because she knew she would never see us again. My dad hadn't seen her since he was aged 20. My Polish grandfather died the year I was born. He had worked in a bank before the war and my father's family were middle class. They owned a house in the country with horses, chickens and lambs. Also a town apartment which was built into the castle walls. Which my granddad used to stay at when he went to work in the city. My grandmother was Austrian. Her name was Maria. My grandfather's name was Michael. My dad was born in Tarnapol, which isn't far from the capital Warsaw. During the War and in the Summer my Gran and Granddad were put to work in the fields of Siberia and unfortunately he had an accident falling off a cart and broke his neck. Dad said he was never the same but he survived only to die just before I was born. I never met my uncle Stanley who was the youngest of the boys. Aunty Sophie was the only girl and the youngest of the five children.

Mum and dad first taught me my thirst for knowledge. Dad was always repairing or inventing things. He loved photography. Once he invented a bed not unlike the one Michael Jackson used to sleep in.

My mother always used to complain at the state of her bedroom because it was littered with film projectors and all sorts of repair work he was doing on TVs and radios etc. Him not ever having a garage or shed of his own which he would have loved.

Dad was highly intelligent and before the war struck and raped Poland he desired to go into the priesthood. This was never to be accomplished and I am grateful he went on to produce and give life to me.

He spoke three languages but unfortunately we never learned to speak Polish unlike my cousins who's first language was Polish. I am quite ashamed I do not speak it.

He had major emotional issues of abandonment and memories of trauma and anxiety. Some soldiers are so traumatized they cannot speak of what they have experienced. My father spoke often of his experiences and we watched the holocaust on television which sometimes used to make my stomach churn and my blood coil.

I am of the opinion that psychiatry and the way mad people have been treated throughout history is worse then any holocaust.

Dad remembers weddings and dances and hot wonderful summers in Poland before the war. Poland had a good economy and was not a poor country. It had resources that is why Hitler invaded her. The Polish people remained occupied for many years after the war. Until Leif Weiwenza formed an uprising and they were liberated. They have been free for 30 years now I think and are part of the common market now. It is nice to meet Polish people working here in my town.

Dad used to bring fruit and nuts home with him as treats. He used to take me into Piccadilly and the market. Buy me hot chestnuts from a barrow. Mum and dad would take us to see Walt Disney films like 'Snow White' and 'Bambi'. And dad once took me to see Eddie Calvert a wonderful trumpet player at the Manchester Palace. As children we used to goto the zoo at Bellevue. And were fascinated with the flea circus. Also there was a huge fairground there. Sometimes we would go see a pantomime. We would all go to the cinema on a Saturday afternoon for the matinee. When older we would watch Laurel and Hardy and Buster Keaton on a Saturday morning followed by Swap Shop with Noel Edmunds. The Marx Brothers were our favourites and Dad loved Charlie Chaplin but used to work on Saturday mornings in the cellar cutting out parts of handbags from leather pieces to be sewn up and riveted the following week.

Mum's family were strong working class salt of the earth people. Grandad was a rope splicer and travelled the country to earn his crust. Gran had eleven children. I do not know how many are still alive today because as families tend to go I have lost touch. All of my aunts and uncles have done well and my cousins. And one cousin used to play rugby for England. My Gran once had a shop and was an excellent cook. The children like most children in those days would all have their jobs and take care of their younger siblings. Mum talked about how they would sit at the table on a Sunday and play cards. When Mark was in hospital one time for six months my mum came and stayed with me. My Mum me and my son Lee who was then 8 or 9 used to play cards and he was excellent at it. With the little money we had we used to entertain him with board games and card games because he didn't have access to videos or at that time computer games. Not until later.

My aunty Cath was the aunt I had most contact with. She never married because she once had an affair with a married man who would not leave his wife for her so she never bothered with men after that. She was lovely. She used to buy toys for all the children in the family and that was a lot. Even for my lee.

My mum was working in a textile mill on the looms when she met my dad who got a job there. Her family were against her marrying him because he used to become suspicious and was lurking outside her home watching her suspecting she had another man once. Her family didn't like that because she was a good living girl.

During the times when Dad used to hit on Mum then Gran did her best to put a stop to it but he threw her out into the street and told her never to return and interfere again. Once I remember before we left Lister Street Mum tried to leave dad but at that time it was very difficult for a woman to survive on her own and raise her children and there were four of us. I remember she told me how she had turned to Gran and asked if she could come live with her but Gran said she had made her bed and had to sleep in it. She would not take in four children and a daughter who had made the terrible mistake of marrying a foreigner.

My mother was a typical 1950's lady who expected a nice home in which she would spend her time and to have a husband who provided her with the money for this lifestyle.

During the fifties there were the rag and bone men who came into the street with a horse and cart selling balloons in exchange for old rags, which were always supplied by mum. When her dolly tub packed up and clothes washing was increased mum used to go to the wash house to do her weekly wash. The laughter and banter of these women as they washed was rich. She did work outside the home once we were all in school and my brother and sister in nursery. She worked as a presser in a dress making factory, the same factory I would approach for free off cuts of cloth so I could sew dresses and outfits by hand for my doll. I wanted to be a fashion designer when I grew up.

Mum was sent for at work one day which was an emergency. Janet and David had locked themselves in the nursery bathroom and set the taps on full. They had caused a flood and the fire brigade had to be called out. The fireman had to climb up his ladder and get in through a window. They were inseparable and up to constant pranks.

Dad had several jobs. Once he worked nights for Dunlops and he became suspicious somebody was going to poison him in his tea. He got paranoid. But he has not suffered from acute madness like me, my brother and uncle Marion.

My uncle Marion settled in this country also after the war and married Mary a Polish girl. Who I adored. They had a boy and two girls who are still alive and live here. And my cousin Terry is very much like her mum and we keep in touch. I love her very much. Marion was younger than dad and during the war he suffered from immense trauma which caused his madness later in life. He was hospitalized and drugged. And once on a visit to his home he was suffering from Akithisea and I advised he take the side affect tablets which helped him. But I did not know the truth about it all then and what I was suffering myself. And how these drugs and their terrible side effects are masked by other medication, such as side effect tablets.

When we were children my brothers and sister and I used to sneak off and on the steam trains and travel into the countryside off on adventures. Packing sugar butties and bottles of orange juice we roamed into orchards and went scrumping for apples and picking blackberries. We would sometimes bring this fruit home for mum to bake an apple or blackberry pie. She had no cooker and just had a little hob with two rings and a small oven. What an experienced cook she was to prepare a roast chicken dinner for six with baked desert and custard to follow every Sunday on such a tiny appliance. Our terraced house had no inside bathroom and there was an outside loo which was freezing in the winter time and smelly during the summer months. Bath times were in a steel bath by the open fire. The eldest in first the youngest last of the children. Mum and dad on their own. Mum had to boil the water on the fire and fill up the bath this way. Bubble bath wasn't around and just soap was the norm. Talcum powder to dust down was a nice luxury.

They weren't the good old days not by a long chalk but I don't remember feeling particularly down or depressed and basically throughout the trauma there was indeed happiness. We had little but knew of little and didn't expect or desire much. We enjoyed the simple things in life and appreciated this for what it was and weren't striving for something better all of the time. We had to live with what money we had and if your dad and mum didn't work you literally starved or went into care. So we were happy to get what we were given and didn't feel neglected or unprivileged. Why?

Because we were part of a community and we were all in the same boat. Now the nuclear family is isolated with no extended family members with only television and the media as an outlet into the world. Those who do have extended family are lucky and thrive. But there are many living isolated and lonely lives today.
So the bad old days have improved for many. Certainly for myself. Still for all of the classes in today's society there are new and numerous problems in living.

Chapter 9 TRAUMA

Around the time I was aged 10 ½ mum began to suffer from heavy periods and as is the norm gynaecologists recommend a hysterectomy. So, mum had to go into hospital for this major operation.

Us children were sent to an orphanage run by nuns in Bury on the outskirts of Manchester which was surrounded by countryside. It must have been the Spring and the Summer of 1961.

This was a particularly traumatic time for all of us. Recently my brother Chris told me he remembered some of the abuse he suffered at the hands of the older children. According to what he recollects he was made to line up with the other kids whilst the older ones hit them on the back of the legs with a cricket bat. By then Chris was a cripple having contracted polio when he was 4 years old. So this was a particularly cruel act done to him.

I remember one time rescuing my baby sister from the others who were tossing her in the air inside a cardboard box. Janet recalls how the nuns tried to separate us all. But when the chance arose we used to wonder off into the countryside by ourselves. We used to take off for the day and spend hours wondering around the fields and country lanes. Janet fell into a cow pat one day when disembarking from a stile. She said a nun washed her hair and really was rough with her and it hurt. My memories of that time are brief. I remember each night at bedtime we were given a warm beaker of milk. We all had our own beakers and toothbrushes with our names on.

We were given a sixpence on a Saturday to spend at the tuck shop on sweets.

I know I have blotted a great deal of my memories about that time out of my head. Janet recollects how David used to lie in bed at night when an owl in the tree outside his bedroom window used to hoot and kept him awake and frightened. He used to wet the bed which he never did at home and the nuns used to beat him for it.

When we experience trauma, that is to say when we are in a situation where there is no way out and it is intolerable the mind goes into fight or flight mode. Our memories are absorbed by the part of the brain called the hippocampus which passes it onto and stores it in the amygdala which is like our small brain within our brain. The memory of a traumatic experience like this is absorbed by the hippocampus but isn't stored in the amygdala and it becomes broken up into the body and that memory is forgotten. Then we disassociate but the feeling of that memory can be triggered by our senses later on in life.

I feel that it was my childhood trauma that has gone on to affect me in adult life and does make me go mad and is the cause of my madness.

It usually starts off my you wondering about relationships and how you have failed in them. How you fit into your community and the outside world. Then for me I started, because reality was so difficult, to start to day dream. I day dreamed all day from when I awoke to all day at work to last thing at night. I day dreamed my life where I wanted it to be with the people I wanted to be in it. I still find myself day dreaming about someone or people or something I want to happen. But when I am not mad I can snap out of it and realise that I am just dreaming.

Then this daydreaming turns into delusions which are like dreaming completely and nobody can tell you that they are not real because you are living in them. You are living your dreams. Psychosis is like when you are dreaming and the rapid eye movements stops and you go into deep sleep. This is what psychosis is. Being in a sleep state whilst being awake.

When I was 17 I suffered from suicidal ideation and severe anxiety and insomnia. But I don't remember being in psychosis or being delusional until after I was prescribed Lebrium.

When mum arrived at the orphanage to collect us she looked well, smartly dressed and a picture of health. She had convalesced with her family.

A little while later dad tried to set up a handbag making business and rented some rooms in Bury New Road. One day mum was taking us four children there to meet up with dad and because I had been before I ran ahead by myself.

When I got there Geoff the man who owned the shop downstairs was out so I went up to the rooms. I ran upstairs and there was a man who looked quite ugly but was well dressed. He had a hair lip and wore a suit and trilby. He held a piece of paper in his hands and said he had brought a letter for my dad. Would I like to read what it said. So a curious 11 year old that I was I went to look. Then this ugly man reached down to me and started to fondle my young sprouting breasts. I jerked free of him and said that I would tell my dad what he did and my dad would beat him up.

Of course I ran back to mum and blurted out what had happened. This caused a major row with my mum and dad but a few days later dad was doing business with and laughing and joking with this man.

Dad said he had to put food on the table.

Then came one of the highlights of the year for us children. November 5th Guy Fawkes Night. We loved bonfire night even though some of the kids used to throw bangers and you used to have to get out of the way quick. It was a chance to stay up late and I remember we used to bake hot potatoes in the large fires and the fireworks dad used to light up were wonderful.

The fires were comforting at the same time we used to sit by them excited and lost in the merriment of it all. The black nights and stars in the clear winter skies above added to the fun. Songs like Twinkle Twinkle Little Star were sung.

Toffee apples were bought from the local shop for sixpence and bowls of apples in water were brought out as a game which was known as 'Bob the Apple'. The idea was you picked up an apple from the bucket of water by your teeth hands behind your back and you simply kept the apple if you succeeded to pick it up.

A couple of weeks before this particular night I went with the other kids in the neighbourhood to collect firewood for the bonfire. Dad said to me that on no account should I go down the alley whilst the boy next door Billy was there. Apparently mum and dad had seen him and a girl from our neighbourhood having sex on the shed roof on one of that Summer's night.

Stubborn and defiant I disobeyed and that night dad beat me to within an inch of my life. I was totally innocent and had done nothing wrong.

Once when I was grown mum and me were on a bus travelling somewhere and she pointed out to me a row of houses. She said that the man who assaulted me owned them and they used to be brothels.

At 11 years of age this gave me my second lesson in where I stood in life and a strong belief in just what some men were capable of including my own father.

In 1962 I left primary school for secondary education. The school I was allocated to was a brand new girls school in Victoria Park. But I wanted to go to Dunstable House because my friends were going there. Dunstable House was an old residential Victorian house that had been transformed into a school. I had numerous arguments with mum about this but being stubborn and a teenager I won.

Our form teacher there was Mrs McDonald. She must have been at least 60 years old and should have been retired. She tied her hair back in a severe bun and she dressed plainly and was plump in stature. She wore glasses which she peered down through the end of her nose. Her breath smelled of tea which she drank by the gallon.

I remember one time after a lesson about etiquette she brought in some of her old whale-bone corsets to teach us young girls. They must have been at least a size 20. Her motive was that we learn how to wear the correct undergarments which gentile ladies would wear. This to a class of young 13 year olds who were all a size 8 or 10.

One Christmas time she brought us all in a present. She placed this mystery gift all wrapped up in tissue paper onto her desk and lovingly began to unwrap it. She had our attention. When she finally opened this wonderful 'gift' we saw that it was a brand new state-of-the-art cowhide leather strap.

Before the holidays and when she was out of the room we got together and hid it behind one of the cupboards along with the corsets. Ma McDonald never did find them. When the school was being shut down ready for demolition I cannot imagine the surprise somebody must have had when they were found hidden behind the cupboard.

During the 1960's I made friends with a young girl a little older than me. She lived across the street opposite to us. Mary and me used to sit on our doorstep of a summer evening and listen to radio Luxembourg and radio Caroline on my little tranny.

During that time the domestic violence at home had become more and more aggressive. In one vicious bout mum accused Mary's family of being depraved poverty stricken dirty people. That the Maloney children were neglected and never looked after. That the Irish were like that. Mary had alopecia in her scalp and mum said that this was caused through her hair not being washed and that she used too much hair spray.

Listening to this and the impact of mum's words made me pick an unprovoked fight with Mary the next day in school. Then her best friend Sheilah sought me out and beat me up in the school toilets.

Also I verbally attacked Christine who lived on our street because of what mum had said about her family being no good Irish who had brothers bringing home the bacon. I remember the look of disbelief on Ma McDonald's face. There was no explanation for my behaviour.

I know now what mum in her desperation was saying in anger. That she hated the poverty she was witnessing around her and yes Christine and her family had a better way of life because her menfolk were in work and dad was struggling to bring home money to feed us. There was no DHSS or unemployment benefit for families to fall on back then and if your parents didn't work you starved or were sent into care.

Mum and dad worked hard all their lives but just could not earn enough money to live comfortably. They ran a handbag business. Dad had his wide interests and hobbies on the cheap. And mum was an avid reader belonging to 4 large libraries in the City.

When Dunstable House was shut down and I was 13 we were all given places at St .Pius X Comprehensive School. Although by that time I could not produce academic work of any value the experience I had at this school was good.

I enjoyed this school with its airy classrooms and new desks that smelled of pine. It had its own swimming pool and chapel. We were allocated a new school uniform which was grey with a red blouse with a rolled collar. We had a little waistcoat and the jacket was modern. We also had a red jockey cap but nobody wore that.

I picked up domestic science and did well at needlework and cookery. Mum having taught me to knit and sew. One day at the end of term there was a fashion show and I modelled the new dress I had made. I wore my hair in a bob like the 60's singer Sandy Shaw and my figure had grown neat and trim. I used to cut the cardboard centre of toilet rolls in half and clip them under my hair and sleep with them. Then I had my bob the next day. Janet said everybody wanted to know my trick but I wouldn't tell anybody.

I didn't realise it at the time but I was in fact pretty and the ugly duckling was turning into a swan. My sister and brothers were good looking too.

I was good at art. A portrait I did of David MacCullum from the TV programme 'A Man from UNCLE' was hung outside the art class for a year. At that time we were living in rooms in Victoria Park because we had not long been evicted from Lister Street because dad had not paid the £5 rent he felt he should not pay because the landlord did no repairs and the ceiling was leaking in the front bedroom and we all ended up sleeping in the front parlour. People were poor in Lister Street but I would say we probably were the poorest family. This taught me shame and I suppose caused most of my feelings of inferiority along with lack of self confidence. But I grew to be quite an attractive young woman with long brown hair with auburn streaks, hazel green eyes and a trim figure. 34" 26" 34" for most of my young adult years. My husband said I would have made a good glamour model and I have never had any trouble attracting the opposite sex and even now in my senior years this does not prove to be a problem.

At around the time I lived in Victoria Park I was walking down an alley on my way home when I found a magazine on the ground. Curious I started to read its contents and found that it was soft porn. The contents were of a threesome two women and a man and one of the women performed falatio on the man. His cum trickled down from her mouth and onto her breasts. I did not find this repulsive. It did not disgust me or frighten me it just made me extremely curious. I was 14 years old at the time and just discovering my body and masturbation although mum never taught me anything about this and there was no sexual education in schools around that time which would have been about 1965. So I suppose curiosity got the better of me and as I was having lessons in typing at school and dad had bought me a little Remington typewriter I thought I would type out this article and give copies to my friends. Of course mum caught me and I cannot imagine what would have happened if I had distributed copies to my friends. Their parents would have created an uproar with my parents. There might have even been a vigilante against my parents. It was the time of Mary Whitehouse and Enoch Powell. Mary Whitehouse was a staunch moralist and had plenty of media coverage with her outrageous disgust at what can only be described as harmless fun. Today although people are pretty paranoid when it comes to their children and paedophiles and threats to our children of a sexual nature which is warranted in most of today's societies, we have come a long way in accepting our sexualities. Although I feel that sex is sometimes used to sell products and sometimes women are demeaned in the process.

Recently during a hospital admission my last I hope I encountered a really nice lady who had experienced quite a great deal of abuse during her childhood. Her husband had a severe medical condition and she was responsible for looking after him and her three children. She could not have sex with her husband that gave her any satisfaction. My friend had a strong sexual urge and was on the verge of having an affair with another patient who had told her nothing but lies about himself. Of course her husband intervened and requested she be moved so she ended up hundreds of miles away from home in the Priory where we met. I know that psychiatric medications can cause a lessening of labido but they can also cause an increase in labido too. So she had quite a struggle in her life.

One Saturday night Dan a very handsome young nurse was on night duty on our ward and it was like a rooster had been let loose in the hen house. All of us girls were flirting with him and I of course was very attracted to him. My friend asked him out and we laughed and joked about it all. Then we were discussing how being without a sexual partner for whatever reason was just as difficult for women as it was for men and she suggested there should be a magazine so we could look at handsome men. The equivalent of Playboy only for girls.

Recently I had an email from Feminista UK a feminist organization based in London founded by Kat Banyard who wrote The Equality Delusion. The email informed me that because of the constant campaigning of Feminista the magazine NUTS was being taken down off the shelves of large supermarkets. NUTS they have demonstrated against saying how the images of women in the magazine de-humanize women as sexual objects. That is a wonderful victory. Most women I asked about would they be interested in an equivalent magazine for women said they wouldn't. Why? Because we are not reared to de-humanize men as sexual objects. And ask any man would they like their daughter to become a prostitute or to model in the nude suggestively they would say "No!".

In my early 20s the second Women's Movement or as we were nicknamed by the media Women's Lib came about. I used to meet up with some of the girls and go on demonstrations. It was really good for a while for me. And now I wish that I had a friend who was a feminist like me. So I suppose you could say I was an activist of sorts for a while.

When I was 14 I had a boyfriend. He was from the boy's school opposite. The boys used to peer from their hall windows from the boy's school opposite through to our hall windows at us girls having dancing lessons wearing simply red t shirts and large navy blue knickers. We hated those lessons.

This was a time when kissing and cuddling was a welcomed introduction to adulthood. Steve and I wasted no time in doing this every chance we could get.

At that time the BBC recorded the pop music programme Top of the Pops in a street round the corner from our school. Some of us girls used to play hooky on a Wednesday afternoon and hang around outside the dressing rooms hoping to get a glimpse of the stars.

Once there was a person who appeared behind the frosted glass of one of the dressing room windows. I climbed onto the sill trying to see through the clear part at the top. This person and I both moved slowly up together on either side and when we got to the clear part of the window I saw it was Peter Noon from Herman's Hermits. He made a funny face as if the say 'ugly' and I fell back down laughing out loud to my friends.

Another time we chased Peter and Gordon to a local garage where they were filling up their red MGB with petrol and we got their autographs. Also once my friend Denise and I were let into Top of the Pops and were filmed dancing in our school uniform. Peter Asher was the brother of Jane Asher who used to go out with Paul McCartney.

Once the headmistress got wind of this it was put a stop to.

Steve and I became Mods. He had a scooter with mirrors and fur on its aerials. Our friend Nick was Hungarian and loved the blues. We used to go see him and sit in his front parlour and drink tea and play his 48 and 78 vinyl records.

By that time my family had moved to a two storey 3 bedroomed flat in Whalley Range.

Once in the middle of the night during summer Steve, Nick and I snook out and walked for miles down the deserted city streets laughing and joking about. Nobody ever found out but it was just innocent fun and we didn't get drunk or take drugs.

One night after Steve and I were petting heavily at the bus stop I missed my last bus home. Steve took me back to his house where his mum was asleep upstairs with her boyfriend. He laid out the sofa cushions on the floor and we sat and ate oranges and talked all night. In the early hours we attempted to start up the car and woke Steve's mum and boyfriend up. Her boyfriend drove me home and luckily Steve and I both escaped being punished.

Chapter 10 SUICIDE

When I was 16 and had finally left school to work as an office junior in the City. Which was a good start to working life, attending Fielden Park College on one day release to study shorthand and English language, Steve asked me to marry him.

Mum persuaded me not to do it saying Steve would amount to nothing only being an Irish Navvy and that I was too young. I could do much better for myself.

I took my first overdose then and toyed with cutting my wrists with a razor blade.

Steve and I had been going out for two years and I ended the relationship.

It was around the time I first toyed with the idea of suicide that my mother had no choice but to take me to the family GP. He prescribed what GP's always prescribe to newcomers suffering from what is described as mental health problems, he prescribed Lebrium. I was told to go home and take the tablets. They made me spaced out and sleepy.

It was obvious to anybody that as a young teenager I was suffering not from some illness but from immense psychological issues all relating to my childhood. I know that I was beginning to explore my sexuality and that relationships with the opposite sex were becoming a major point in my young life.

My mother had instilled in me that sex outside marriage was a bad thing, especially as it might lead to an unwanted pregnancy. But in the late 1960's early 70's the contraceptive pill was brought onto the market. So this gave women a certain amount of sexual freedom however also causing other problems.

What I needed badly at the age of 16 wasn't a pill to pop, but lessons in sexual education. And advice from someone sound about relationships and just how they should work. My mother seemed not to know let alone was willing to help me with these matters. She herself was and remained sexually frustrated most her married life.

It is so clear to me now that all what I witnessed as a small child, the domestic violence and the loss of my uncle and abuse in the orphanage then my molestation by the brothel owner had manifested into emotional turmoil for me when I came to end my relationship with my boyfriend at the age of 16.

This was no disease or illness this was a normal reaction to trauma and abuse.

I recovered and found myself another job this time in a solicitors office, but I had known what it was like to become withdrawn. I felt somehow so different from other people. I was well capable of doing my job but somehow relationships with the other girls were strained. I found myself another boyfriend but did not have sexual intercourse with him either and this fizzled out.

I was convinced I had cancer of the womb. I felt extremely isolated and alone with only mum to confide in. She again took me to the family GP and mentioned I might need an internal examination.

Reassuring she said she would stay in the examination room with me. Whilst examining me the doctor with his back to mum leered down looking at me and he carried out the procedure like that of a sexual act.

Mum said to me later that Ashworth had told her I had not had intercourse before and was still a virgin but that it probably wasn't for the want of trying. She seemed content with that.

A few years later he attempted to molest my young sister and she slapped his face. Mum made me believe because I hadn't done the same somehow I was to blame for what he did.

I carried that around inside me for a long time and of course she wasn't a bad mother because she had allowed it to happen in front of her to her teenage daughter?

Before she died I tackled her with this over the telephone accusing her that she should have changed doctors and that I actually believed I had cervical cancer. Apparently she shook and trembled on the other end. Sometimes people don't like to face the truth about their actions. My father made me feel as though I should never have done that to her.

It was abuse that caused and has continued to cause my madness, which has blighted me most of my life.

There has never been any doubt in my mind that I am different from other people. Long before I understood about madness I understood this. To be mad is different.

My madness reaches many heights. Many heightened states of reality. It can be harmful and life threatening when you hear voices criticizing you constantly telling you just how bad you are and that you are probably even evil. My particular voices have never goaded me into stabbing or violently hurting someone. I very rarely act on them but I have on a couple of instances in the past. Not really doing much harm to anyone. If nothing else attempting to harm myself.

Paranoia is frightening. You imagine there is somebody or some people out to get you. Once my husband thought the nurses on the ward were going to throw him in a cellar and eat him alive. I can't imagine anything as frightening as that. Because it is real and you are living this reality at the time. Along with my voices paranoia is a very frightening experience.

Then there is the icing on the cake – delusions! Delusions can be either terrifying or a wonderful trip. Unfortunately most of mine are frightening, but they aren't always. With delusions you enter a different world where your life and who you are change completely. You forget your old self and life. This new life and the events in it are and become reality however absurd it takes hold, it seems real. It is kind of like taking part in a play or film. Maybe you are famous or the FBI or CIA are out to get you or want you as an exceptionally important person to work for them. You witness yourself being discussed on the 9 o'clock news. Everything, all of the train of events take place. But the reality is nothing much is happening or has changed. You are dreaming.

This can be frightening or an adventure depending on how your imagination whips up the nature of the delusion.

Psychosis is like being in a sleep state whilst awake, then losing complete touch with reality and going into sleep mode still awake. Psychosis is the most dangerous because it can get you hurt.

I never experienced any of these symptoms before I was prescribed the psychiatric drug Lebrium. This then caused a chemical imbalance in my brain and led to me lead a life embroiled in the psychiatric system.

There is a stage when you are young when you anguish over the fact that you are so extremely different than others. And even understanding madness like I do now sometimes the anguish is there. When for instance I am abused by others because of it. Either by stigma or someone prejudiced has found out I go mad.

Now in my senior years I no longer feel inferior because I enter into other worlds and into other states of reality purely by myself without alcohol or social drugs. I know I am different but I also know I am not inferior because of this. I know others aren't either. I know I go mad because of childhood trauma and sexual abuse. But I never went psychotic or suffered delusions before being prescribed psychiatric medication.

Freud was so right to relate much of our behaviour to sex. We are sexual beings and the intricacies of our sexual drives are powerful.

We become sexual at a young age but for adults to take sexual advantage of an immature young child is wrong. But we do become sexual even as a baby. When this sexuality is abused our sexual lives become distorted and the unconscious cannot reason with the conscious then madness can and most commonly does occur.

For a long time women have been forced to suppress their sexuality. For monogamist relationships most people are unhappy sexually or would sometimes like to explore. You could say that variety is the spice of life for both sexes. This can go for every day things like diet and you could say for our sex lives too. Sometimes the same old partner becomes boring. This is why so many marriages break up,not because people fall out of love but because they need variety in their sex lives. For others familiarity and security are a turn on. Some people simply love their partners and sex comes secondary to their relationship. Everybody is different. Some like regular Sunday roast dinners some like to eat out.

When I was 18 I joined the Queen Alexander's Nursing Corps. I did my basic training at Aldershot for 8 weeks. I have never been so fit in my life before. Then I was posted to Catterick in Darlington, where married men were on the prowl and of course being pretty I got enticed and seduced by one lance corporal. I decided because this was happening to most of my friends I didn't like the army and it wasn't for me. I lost my virginity to him. He wanted to leave the army and his wife and children and marry me. But I decided to end it because I didn't want to be a marriage breaker.

Then because I so loved the nursing side to it I got a job as a pupil nurse at Wythenshawe Hospital in Manchester.

Although I had problems splitting up from this married man I did well in school and came first in my exams. I met up with an old school acquaintance. We ventured out for a night on the town. Sometime during that evening for whatever reason she thought she would slip some drugs into my drink. I became totally high and we all ended up sleeping with some guys, although I was too high even to come down for the sexual act. The next day not knowing just why I had behaved that way I was ashamed and didn't turn into work. The matron sacked me at the same time asking questions about Annmarie. I found out later that Annmarie had been stealing drugs from the wards and using them for her own gain.

Some years later she turned up in my life again and I felt befriended by her. She persuaded me to join her in sharing a flat with her and a Swedish girl and so eager for my independence I agreed and moved in. I became involved with the boy downstairs but to me the relationship meant nothing and was casual. Then out on the town one night I met Colin Terret who was a DJ at a club we went in. He was the younger brother of Ray Terret who was a famous celebrity DJ around Wythenshawe and Manchester. I fell madly for him. I started an affair with Colin and during our times together he told me about his death wish.

I then was neurotic at times and very insecure. Sometimes I would have outbursts. Also there became a big issue with me and this other boy splitting up. Apparently he lost his job and I had told him I would be his girlfriend when in actual fact I felt nothing for him. Annmarie told Colin and he finished with me. Except he didn't tell me to my face and this hurt. Some years later when I was engaged to Mark his mum told me that Colin had been found dead at his nightclub and had hung himself. Just like he said he was going to. You could say I loved Colin.

I remember Annmarie at school and during the art exam how the teacher said we had to paint in colours to gain a good grade and Annmarie whilst I was thinking what exactly to paint goaded all the other girls into using up the coloured paints so I had to paint in black and white. I painted a scene of a gondola in Venice but only came 6th even though I was the best artist in my form.

I have had numerous psychotic and paranoid delusional breakdowns during my life and most of that time I have gone blindly through not knowing what it was exactly that I suffered from. This blindness made it even harder to bare and I felt isolated.

When I was 21 I decided to travel abroad and got myself a job as an au pair. It was with a lovely Italian family in Naples and I adored their little boy Enzo. Enzo had a younger brother named Cico but he thought I was stupid because I couldn't understand his Italian and this three year old couldn't speak English. Rosaria and Genaro had spent a few years in Seattle in America previous to when I went to work for them. So Enzo spoke fluent English. I had a wonderful time and spent 6 weeks in Capri in a villa. Although I was not quite myself. I fell in love with a navigation pilot named Genaro but he turned out to be a real louse. I slept around quite a lot and had many a sexual encounter with the young Italian boys. Carlo was one such boy and he was exceptionally handsome and nice. We talked over the phone but he sounded strange and I presumed he was taking social drugs so I wouldn't see him. He wanted to go steady. Then months later my friend Lyn who was a nurse by profession explained Carlo was an epileptic and probably had just had a fit or was in fact on medication. I was so sorry.

Then when Enzo went to school I was sent to work for their sister to look after her baby. This woman made me not only take care of the baby but clean his room and wash all his clothes and nappies by hand. Also she didn't feed me and I couldn't afford to feed myself on the wages I earned. So I practically lived on biscuits and the meal I had one day a week on a Sunday at their mothers kept me alive. But I lost weight. I was glad I became a size 10 and clothes were cheap and easy to come by.

Then I became insane once again. I was terribly home sick and wouldn't write home for the money to fly back to the UK. I became delusional and paranoid and imagined her big brute of a husband was going to kill me. That I had found out they were smuggling drugs into Italy from Africa because they had a holiday in Morocco that year and brought back African artefacts.

I climbed out of a small window onto a drain pipe then onto the kitchen balcony. This was 9 stories up and very dangerous. I call this my Emma Peel from the Avengers moment. I shouted down to a group of young people below for help and they came up to the flat. Then I wouldn't let them go until I phoned my friend Lyn who worked for a woman employed by the British Consul. I spent time with Jane and Lyn and Lyn remembered a comment I made about food once whilst with her one day. She was dishing out a meal she had cooked and I commented she got fed real food. Then a doctor was called and I was flown home the next day.

Back to old Blighty and the fog and cold. But I was so glad to be back on British soil and home once again.

Lyn, Rosaria and Jane all wrote to me later, but unfortunately I did not reply. Lyn wanted to meet up back in England. Rosaria wanted to know if I was all right and Jane actually offered me a job working with her children. But I decided not to respond and didn't keep in touch with Lyn.

Chapter 11 DEATH

When I was 23 I had my first admittance to hospital. I was suicidal one day and a health visitor had just visited my younger brother who also was diagnosed with Schizophrenia. After she left David saw the state I was in and asked me if I would like him to call her so I said yes. This started my first interview with a psychiatrist. Like most people I thought these were qualified university educated people and knew everything there was to know about madness. Dr. Thompson my registrar told me he thought it was an illness and could be treated. I was glad that what I suffered from was recognized and was also so hopeful it could be treated. So at first I was glad to believe what a bio-psychiatrist like Dr. Thompson told me.

Then I was admitted where I became friends with Andrew. I spent a few weeks there in hospital and found it a nice place to stay. I didn't mind or see it as an intrusion on my liberty. I went willingly and felt secure to be there.

I was discharged and was OK at home. I found myself work. In one office I met up with Alan and after a brief courtship he asked me to move in with him so seeking my own independence again away from my family home I agreed.

The relationship was good then became strained. I told Alan I became ill but I didn't think he would understand or be sympathetic and he wasn't. I went to the doctor and he gave me something, anti-depressants I think, and this caused me to have adverse effects emotionally. Alan and me argued and I ended up shouting in his face. Later after reading Dr. Breggin this too is a side-affect of some of the drugs. I overdosed and this virtually put an end to the relationship.

Then I woke up one morning after having a bad dream that I found my brother dead. Alan took me to visit home and I talked to David inviting him up to stay once again but he said he was broke and maybe another time. Mum said he had sold all his record collection. I told David to take care of his money. Earlier that year when I had been suffering from my own mental anguish he asked me about the medication which he had been taking for years and even then I said I thought it didn't work and was no good.

A week later I was walking home from work and my dad and his next door neighbour were waiting for me outside our flat. Dad explained David was quite ill and would I like to go see him. I said I needed to change and we had to wait for Alan to come home and dad said quietly I should put on something black to wear. I couldn't make sense of it. Then we waited for Alan to come home from work and we all drove back to Manchester. On the way Alan said I should be brave.

When I got there Mum and Janet were crying. I couldn't understand and then dad told me David was dead. That he had hung himself outside on his bedroom balcony. Of course I was beside myself and when Alan said I should consult God I denounced a God who could allow such a terrible thing to happen. My baby brother dead because his life wasn't worth living any more. I blamed my dad.

I now know that what probably made David kill himself was the fact that he was taking psychiatric medication. This and the fact he suffered from suicidal ideation anyway probably pushed him over the edge. He was missing my sister and they were extremely close. Also David was the last one at home and he had just finished with a girl he was in love with.

Then there was a bad time where mum and dad couldn't afford to pay for the funeral costs and were desperate financially. Even if David had been insured they wouldn't have paid out for suicide.

Nevertheless they turned to the Polish church and the Combatants paid for David's funeral which was so good. There was a Polish singer and of course the service was all in Polish and the church was lovely decorated with beautiful flowers. Beforehand we all went to see David at the funeral parlour it was the second time I had seen a dead body. This time someone close who I loved. Mum held his hand and warmed it. He was cold. I still miss him today and always will. I wish I could console myself that one day we would meet again. But I am simply of the belief I do not know.

For a short time his poems were read out at the local library. He wrote a poem about me called Sad Lady. I think my dad has copies somewhere.

I picked myself up and got a job in the city and started to commute. Then I decided this relationship Alan and I had was going nowhere so I ended it. Alan told me he hadn't loved me but said I would probably make someone a good wife.

Chapter 12 LIFE

Then on a Spring day in 1977 I admitted myself on to Ward P10 and on that day met Mark. The love of my life.

I thought nothing more of this handsome young man who I met on that day and his wonderful beautiful eyes. Until I saw him on my ward kicking a door open. I asked this peculiar woman about him and she said she had heard Mark was dangerous. But of course he wasn't.

Then that summer I was sat out on the bench and Mark came up beside me and asked if I would go out with him. I said I didn't think manic depression and schizophrenia would mix but would consider it once we left hospital.

One day someone came up to me from his ward and said Mark liked me and that he had the flu and was quite poorly. So when Andrew and I were walking around the grounds I picked a red rose and went to see Mark who was sat head down depressed. I spoke to him but he didn't answer so I placed the rose at his feet.

I asked Andrew about him and he said that he thought Mark was OK.

Then before I knew it he was everywhere, everywhere I went he followed. Like a faithful dog following its master. He was even there when I woke in the morning peering over me in my room. I remember telling the ward sister to stop this man following me and coming into my room whilst I was in bed.

Somehow they gave him a room a few doors down to mine on my ward. He had a sugar bowl milk jug and teapot for his cups of tea. And had brought his records and player in also.

He was just there and then somehow I wanted to be with him and being with him was exciting, I had never known anyone who was manic before and the energy that exuded from him was intoxicating. He was vibrant, very popular and very funny. I didn't fall for Mark straight away but slowly, slowly I fell in love with him. There have been times when I have hated him but deep down I never stopped loving him.

To begin with before I started to go out with him he left a photograph of himself on my bed saying to his brother if she rips it up she doesn't like me. I didn't but I remember telling Idris that if he loved Mark tell him to keep away from me because I was trouble.

We became inseparable and he took me to the pub where we drank St. Clements a non-alcoholic beverage. We were both on Modecate injections which gives your skin an adverse affect with the sun and you burn. We used to put cream on ourselves we bought from the Ian Snow shop in the village. It smelled lovely. Then on my birthday he bought me three tiny little hearts and stars to put on my key ring. I kept them for so many years then lost them one time in hospital.

He introduced me to his mother who I think hoped he wasn't serious about me. Because she knew how difficult a time we would have both being diagnosed with a mental illness.

Then when we were both discharged Dr. Thompson found me a place in a halfway house because I desperately wanted a place of my own. Mum and dad continued to argue and row most days of their married life together. There was really no peace at home to be had. But they were quiet and subdued when David died and the atmosphere was awful. They were getting ready to move out and into a council flat in Wythenshawe. Still quite not myself I stayed at this terrible half way house and was expected to sort out all my finances with the DHSS and job centre. Never having done this before and having to find a doctor I asked Ashworth the family GP who molested me and he said no as he was leaving the practice. It wasn't so much what he said but the way he said it. This was a blow too because I hadn't known any other GP at the time.

This was near to Christmas time and I went to live back home not being able to stand the awful half way house. I never used to dress or wash until Mark came to visit me in the evenings. I was so glad when he left that he had been to see me. One Saturday afternoon because I was behaving aloof he asked me if he should go and not see me again and I was feeling so bad about not being myself I said maybe he should. So he left and thinking I would not see him again I couldn't bare it so I sent my dad to chase after him and he came back. The strain of the move on me would have been horrendous so Mark asked his mum if I could stay with them. She didn't like me I think because my mum had told her I had had a lot of men and as Mark hadn't had many women it would not work out between us. How could she say that about her own daughter to a future mother in law? She was looking out for my welfare in her way I think?

Staying at Mark's was like being in seventh heaven. Her home was so cosy and comfortable. It wasn't a wealthy home by no means but so cheerful and bright. I slept in a huge oak double bed and her white cotton sheets were crisp and fresh. Her cooking was good too. She baked and we had desert after every meal.

She went away over Christmas for a couple of days to stay at a friends and Mark and I took this opportunity to sleep together. It felt so right. We had known each other for 6 months by then. He was prescribed 1,000mgs lithium three times a day and couldn't get an erection. But it didn't stop me from having an orgasm and he was satisfied too. But he had problems with this all our married life.

Then on Xmas Eve he asked me to marry him and he bought me an engagement ring. Afterwards my mum and dad got allocated a flat just a few streets away from where Mark lived so it was easy for us to see each other. We both went back to work and I got a job at a solicitors who used to have some celebrities on their books. Godley and Creme and also there was a song which got to number one in 1977 which was about Lowry the artist called 'Matchstick Men and Matchstick Cats and Dogs' sung by Brian and Micheal. I met those two singers too. But I didn't get along with the girls as I had plenty of free time and they were hard pressed to work.

Mark and I used to have sex in the evenings in his room. He couldn't get an erection but that didn't stop me having an orgasm just by lying on top of him and he too enjoyed himself. This was because he was prescribed 1,000mg of lithium each day. We found out later that they could have poisoned him. Such is the toxicity of the drug. I told him to stop taking it which he did and our sex life improved immensely.

Mark was a very spiritual person. He believed in Jesus. He had telepathic experiences with people. He also had an out of body experience and a vision of Jesus.

Mark seemed to have had a good life before meeting me. He had boating holidays on the Norfolk Broads and camping holidays. He was close to his older sister. And his mum.

His parents were fairly strict. One time he and a friend from school went to watch 'A Cold Beer in Alice' at the pictures and he watched it twice so got home at 11pm that night. His father was there to confront him and took him straight up to the bath where he nearly drowned Mark. His dad was so angry that he had worried his mum so. Also Mark suffered abuse at school. He was bright and top of his class but the teachers wouldn't move him to a higher class because he didn't go to church on a Sunday. It was a Roman Catholic school.

But there was more to what Mark suffered as a child. He didn't tell me or couldn't recall the real abuse. We never discussed or talked about it. He had simply blotted it out of his mind. Now after giving this a lot of thought I realize what could have happened to my Mark was that he was probably sexually abused by a Catholic priest in church. This would have been enough for my Mark to bury such a trauma and in fact cause his mania at the age of his early twenties when he basically became properly sexually active.

He left school at 15 and did a gardening apprenticeship with Wythenshaw Parks for 6 years. He became a foreman landscape gardener. Mark used to work his men hard but he also worked hard himself. And the men respected Mark. When his dad died he lost all loyalty to the council and took his men to the pub for a drink on a Friday afternoon on pay day. His bosses didn't like this.

 When he was 24 years old he started to become down then very happy and couldn't understand the reason he felt so good. Nothing out of the ordinary had changed yet he seemed excited and very happy. When he was 23 he went too fast around a bend in his new Mini Metro and the car rolled over and almost hit a tree. He banged his head badly but wasn't concussed and never went to hospital for treatment. He started to suffer with depression when he was 24. He would lie in bed all day. His mother used to leave the house and slam the door behind her. She couldn't deal with the fact that one of her men folk wouldn't go to work. Then he would go into mania and into orbit.

When he was aged around 28 he became very manic one night and took off on his motor bike with no leathers on or crash helmet. He rode at speed and imagined he was Jesus Christ and that if he drove through the oncoming roundabout he would save the world. So he did just that missing the tree in the middle. He staggered injured to the side of the roundabout and two police men in a car were passing and noticed him sat down on the curb. They knew he was injured but couldn't figure out how he got there because they couldn't see the bike which was hidden by shrubs. Then they found it and of course rushed him to hospital where he spent 6 hours in surgery. He had half his bowels removed. All his ribs down his right hand side were broken and his right lung punctured.

When he came round in intensive care he was full of tubes but Mark being high decided he was going to get out of bed and started to walk around. This just after a major operation and all of his ribs were broken down one side of his chest.

The doctor called his mum and said if they didn't come and remove Mark they would call in the army. Poor mum Watmough must have been in a state to hear this. Then they admitted him to Withington Psychiatric Unit and his career started with psychiatry also. The nurses there didn't tend his wound and his dad used to come in and do that.

At one time when high he went to the casino and knew just what would come up on the roulette wheel. He won £300 that night.

Another time his mum was in bed and heard him talking to the priest down stairs. She went down and saw in the kitchen Mark sitting by himself. There was no priest and Mark had been imitating his voice.

Mark had had around two or three admittances also before we met. It was sheer coincidence that we were in the hospital together at the same time.

I said to Mark one day that having sex sneakily in his bedroom with his mum downstairs wasn't fair on her so on the Sunday night he said should we get married. I said when and he said this week. So we did. This was probably the most exciting week of my life. We invited who we could. Arranged the witnesses. Bought my dress. Bought the rings. Hired a car and put a deposit on a luxury flat. Mark got a special licence. He asked me on the Sunday and by the Friday we were married and living together.

Life was good. But Mark wasn't happy at work. Every time he was away in hospital his team of men who he had built up used to get disbanded and this frustrated Mark. Also he felt he wasn't earning enough money. I earned more than him. Although our flat was nice Mark didn't like that either.

I knew how unhappy he was at work so I told him to leave which was a bad move to make. Then he became ill once again. He was admitted and I used to go see him every day. I was talking to him one time and he disappeared. I went looking for him and found him naked on top of a naked woman attempting to make love to her. He told me later that he thought she was me.

I was concerned about medication then. They gave Mark huge doses of medication and were injecting him with Haldol every half an hour. Seeing how this was affecting him I actually thought he was going to die. I demanded to see his psychiatrist and the nurse wouldn't get him so I kicked her in the shins. Then the police were called and I left. Before leaving the grounds I realised I had left behind my shopping bag and that nights dinner so I went back. The nurse and police man were talking. He took one look at me then forced my arm up my back and threw me in a black maria.

This was my first encounter with the police. I spent a night in a cell and then went before the magistrate the next morning. The police man lied about what I did and said. The magistrate was very sympathetic and bound me over for £10.

Then one day when he was better Mark was in the job centre and someone knew a person at the job centre here in Newtown. Mark knew Newtown from when he visited as a child and came to see his uncle Vincent and aunty Mary who lived here. Mary was his mum's sister. They lived in a nice house on top of a hill and Vincent was the Executive Director of the local wool factory. He was also a Free Mason and they paid for his son's education at university. Mark came up fishing as he got older.

The most famous person known in relation to Newtown's history is Robert Owen. Robert Owen was born in Newtown and left for London and his fortune when he was ten years old. He found work in a cotton mill and then had the fortune to own one and then several and he became rich. He became one of the first philanthropists to set up the cooperative movement. And went on to build a small community in Scotland along with a school which was run in quite an inspirational way. There is a statue of him in a little garden here in Newtown and his grave is here because he spent his last years here.

Mark found out there were jobs to be had and a house to go with them so he brought me up to see and went for an interview at one of the factories. I liked Newtown. It was in the March of 1979 and there was a good layer of snow on the ground but it was sunny. I loved the town. It was sleepy then and not much here but I liked that too. The air was so fresh and I loved the hills surrounding the valley and walking along the River Severn which runs through it. I still like Newtown and have lived here ever since.

Mark got the job and we were allocated a house and moved in and he went to work. We didn't have much but his mum helped us out with furniture and my mum with kitchen stuff and curtains and bedding. I had bought one or two items as well. Mark earned good money. In fact a lot for those days. I applied for a job as a nursing assistant at the local hospital but when the Matron interviewing me asked if I had any illness because the nurse I was replacing had been away from work a long time with an illness I had to tell her about my mental health. So like most employers they don't take you on if you tell them. They are led to believe you are totally unreliable in the work force. Which isn't the case. Except I think flexible working hours and days is probably the best for people like me.

But things went terribly wrong when Thatcher became prime minister. Everything in Newtown seemed to close down or fold and there was no work for Mark. Most factories went under.

During the next twelve years we struggled. Before his work stopped I decided to go for a baby knowing that happiness and happiness alone would keep us sane. I got pregnant with Lee who was then born at the cottage hospital on 8th January 1980. We were over the moon and had everything we needed for him.

When Lee was 6 months things started to go terribly wrong and Mark's factory closed down. There was no other work for him. I became insane again and so did Mark. He bought a car and drove me, his mum and Lee back to Withington in Manchester because the hospital in Wales didn't have a mother and baby unit. I stayed there for about 5 weeks whilst Mark was in Denbeigh in North Wales. That was a bad time.

I was delusional and thought Mark's brother was on the roof riding on a motorbike and was after me. At one time I actually thought he had shot me. But I cared for Lee and fed and looked after him. The nurses wouldn't help me with my baby because they knew I had nobody where I lived and Mark did become so ill. So basically they taught me to cope even when not well. And most of the time I coped even though bad until I couldn't any more.

Then I heard from Mark and I said to him "I thought you were dead" he said "I am" and hung up the phone. He told me later he had been on a ward with the criminally insane and at one time was put in solitary into a room which had shit on the walls. All of this for a driving offence when he didn't even have a crash or hurt anyone.

When I was discharged Janet took me to Mark's mum to stay and she helped me cope a lot. Idris took me up to Denbiegh to see Mark. When we met I rushed up to him and threw my arms around him but he hardly responded. Then he was discharged and we went home to Newtown and like so many times in the future to come we picked up the pieces of our lives once more.

Lee is now 34 and I love him so much because he is supportive and caring even though he struggles through with his own personal madness. There were so many times in his childhood he saw either one or both if his parents behaving strangely and he had to be uprooted when both of us became unwell. But this didn't cause his madness.

When he was a young man working as a shop manager his colleague died suddenly and this there was an awful atmosphere in the shop so he left after working there for several years. He had issues of abandonment and issues that had to be dealt with about having two parents who went mad. He started to suffer with extreme anxiety and insomnia and became frightened because of this. Fearing he would go mad one day himself like us. He needed psychotherapy from the onset and talking therapy but instead the GP gave him anti depressants and prescribed a high dose of SSRIs. This brought about his mania. He was never manic before taking these prescribed medications. At the time I hadn't read Breggin and wasn't aware like so many of the harmful toxic affects of these drugs. And the withdrawals and side affects. Otherwise I would have kept him well clear and away from any doctor. Now I have no choice and have to resort to calling the police who ignore me and Lee goes to the police station because he gets deluded. So he ends up on a psychiatric unit and they put on the same ward I was on at the Priory except the male side. And they have him on more drugs now.

He knows the damage that has been done to him. He will be the first to say. But he feels he is compelled to take these medications because even without them he gets manic and delusional the chemical imbalance has already been created in his brain.

There were many times on many occasions when Mark and I became insane. Sometimes individually sometimes at the same time. When this happened we had to send Lee to Mark's sister who always came for him and dropped everything to collect him. So Lee was never in care. She has been quite wonderful.

There were times I broke Mark's heart and he mine. There was one time I broke our vows and had a sexual experience with somebody whilst in hospital and ill. But out of all the breakdowns I had whilst we were married I never strayed. Mark almost strayed once but I stopped it. We stood by each other through thick and thin. He becoming quite manic and spending months in hospital. Once I spent 6 months in there with him not being insane myself. They just thought I couldn't cope on my own. Now I am totally on my own and cope really well!

In 1995 our then psychiatrist offered to help us financially. Mark had previously visited a GP and asked for a six month sick note and to be placed on Family Credit which was a good deal more then the money we were receiving which was the basic Income Support. We were entitled to this by law but this doctor said he couldn't provide the sick notes as this would be illegal. This was the same doctor who when my son was four years old and had pneumonia he couldn't diagnose it. Lee was delirious and I insisted an ambulance be called. I spent two weeks in hospital with him. So we were years without the money we should have been entitled to. This doctor was sacked from the practice eventually.

When Mark did eventually receive Family Credit we went on our first holiday to Butlins at Pawhelli. We took along one of Lee's friends and it was a good break. But we ran out of money and it was self catering so we had to return a day earlier. We were so broke we had no money for milk to make a cup of tea and of course tobacco. But when we arrived home there was a card for my birthday from my sister Janet and in it she enclosed £5 so she literally saved us. And we were able to have a cuppa and buy some food and tobacco to last until pay day. Which was on the following Monday and I had fish fingers and chips in for Lee.

In 1996 John Major brought in Disability Living Allowance and we were allocated the top rate along with extra income support. We became rich compared to how we lived before. It was like winning the lottery. It spiralled Mark into mania once again but after 6 months he recovered and remained sane for 17 years until just before he died.

Mark got his licence back and passed his driving test and we bought our first car. We used to travel out most week's and we met up with the family. We enjoyed long walks at the Elan Valley, Gabowen or even as far afield as Cheltenham. Sometimes we would stay overnight at Maureen's, Idris's or my mum and dads. I remained sane for 4 and half years never having stayed sane for so long. Then I met up with an old patient I knew and at that time her husband left her. She lost custody of her children to her in laws and couldn't even see them or talk to them again.

This came about because she was prescribed Depixol and this increased her libido. She got involved with a drug addict who had a history of abusing children and one day she was having sex with him and locked her two boys outside in her garden. They were crying to come in and a neighbour reported her to social services. So she was given the choice give up this man or give up your children. She wouldn't give up the man.And they were handed over to her in laws who raised them.

 This so distressed me and brought back all the stress and distress I had leaving Lee as he was growing up that I became insane again and was admitted to Telgarth Mid Wales Hospital. The woman herself who was diagnosed schizophrenic like me kept out of hospital for years.

Over the years I have been prescribed many medications and also been given shock treatment. I watched as Mark was given shock treatment and just how he reacted to the anaesthetic which was an awful site to witness. I watched as he became spellbound and not spontaneous and how he wasn't the same man I married. I never stopped loving Mark but around 2004 his chest started to get bad and he was smoking heavy. He wouldn't exercise and liked to spend long journeys in the car. He drank on a regular basis but wasn't violent or aggressive but cordial and good humoured when tipsy and he wanted me to cook rich meals for him, which I did gladly. But then in around 2006 his chest started to get really bad and we started to argue about him smoking and then the arguments led into rows until I wanted to leave. Tried to but had to come back. Then in 2008 I threw him out. I just couldn't watch him kill himself. Also my health was suffering and I couldn't seem to quit the habit either. With what I was witnessing happening to our son and how it devastated me the thought Mark was killing himself over smoking simply because he enjoyed the addiction and the fact once he was gone I would be totally alone to deal with my own condition the abuse of the system and my sons insanity. So I wanted to be left alone in the end.

But there was another reason I ended my marriage to Mark. When I first read Toxic Psychiatry I realised just how true the things that Dr Breggin wrote were. My mother tried in vain to keep me away from doctors and psychiatrists. And when I met Mark he made me believe that she didn't love me because she did this and the right way to go was down the road of medication and with these doctors. So for years I lived down this road with him. Believing I had some sort of brain disease. Suffering all the side affects sometimes not even being able to walk up the stairs. All my adult life I suffered. Because Mark believed in doctors and nurses and these drugs.

He led me to believe my brother and sister didn't love me because they did nothing for me over the years. Janet was living in America. Chris was living in Newcastle upon Tyne which is really hard to get to from Newtown and wasn't in a position to help me. Chris is crippled and his back troubled him so he wasn't able to make the long journey by car to see me. But I drifted apart from my brother although I will always love him and he is a good man.

He stayed at his brothers then his brother's wife Anne who had always been in love with him wanted Mark to move into a flat with her and he wouldn't and realised he missed me. He ended up manic once more and driving on the wrong side of the road during the middle of the night and was admitted to a psychiatric hospital.

I didn't know where he was then found him in Leicester. Made numerous calls and found his car. I ended up owing over £200 to BT but the bill was in Mark's name and I still get threatening letters from debt collectors asking for payment. I give them his current address the Cemetery Poole Road in Newtown.

He was given neuroleptics and consequently because of his bad health his legs and feet swelled up. He was put on the medical side of the hospital. Then homeless he was staying at the housing shelter here in Newtown and was allocated a flat but he didn't want to move in. Alan Davis his CPN admitted him to hospital. He was there for months then one day he called me and told me they said he had cancer. I felt a part of me had died that day. Of course I had him home.

I nursed him the best I could. The MacMillan nurse came to the house. She told Mark what medication he should take and what dosage I should give him. What she didn't tell us is that he was receiving chemotherapy. This made Mark constantly vomit.

For a few months the psychiatric nurse came to the house and gave him injections. Then he stopped coming. Eventually because of the withdrawals Mark became delusional and paranoid. He imagined I was harming him and I actually think he thought I was going to kill him. So he was frightened the last few weeks before he died.

Then after an admittance to hospital for a blood transfusion the specialist told him it had reached his kidneys and that basically he was very ill. Somehow I didn't think and I said I hoped he lived until Christmas but by that time he was insane. He couldn't stop talking and never made sense and couldn't tell me when he needed the toilet. At one time he threw a urine bottle over the sofa. I couldn't cope with him. So he was sent to the hospice who couldn't cope with him either. I was told that he had been playing his music too loud which was a lie because he couldn't get out of his chair to do that. He had become frightened and the nurses at the hospice couldn't cope with that.

So he ended up back in the Psychiatric Hospital and they did their best to give him palliative care. Showing Mark much respect and affection. I visited regularly doing what I could.

He kept saying over and over that the wind would carry him and the angels would get him there. Nobody knew what he meant but sat with him and the social worker I asked Mark did he mean the wind would blow in the sails of the ship and get him there to heaven. And the angels would help get him there. He said relieved "Yes!" I told them later that people who go mad sometimes talk in cryptic sentences but there is a meaning to them so they can tell you what they are saying if you get to know the person and ask them the right questions. Mark used to read books about sailing ships and the Spanish Armada years ago.

Then Lee came one day and we sat beside his bed. He could see by the look in my eyes how sad I was and concerned about him. That he was in fact dying. But he looked at us with fear. Lee helped him sit up and place his pillows as comfortably as he could sit up. I knew he hadn't long so. I asked if I could stay the night on this particular visit but the doctor said no it wasn't hospital policy. Lee and I went home by train then I had a call from the hospital to get back there quick. It was late by this time but fortunately I was able to get a taxi and made it to Mark's bedside. He was then in a coma but I talked to him and felt he could hear me.

I kissed him and told him I loved him. I always had. Then I played the Dubliners his favourite band. He grunted once and I thought what had I done wrong? Then I realised afterwards I was playing the Dubliner's ' I will be a rover no more'. I didn't know he thought I was killing him and what had happened was he cried out. But I loved my Mark and wanted him to be well and drug free without the horrible withdrawals which occur when the anti-psychotics are reduced or stopped abruptly.

Then fluid from his lungs came up into his mouth and he died. He died at 3am on November 30th 2009. Then the nurses drove me home and I told Lee who took it quite well.

We had to go the Shrewsbury to collect the death certificate. Then his body was brought to Newtown. In his open coffin I asked for him to be dressed in his jeans and t shirt. With his denim jacket. In his pockets I place his mobile phone and tobacco and lighter. Either side of him I placed a can of Fosters. Sandals on his feet. Sunglasses in his breast pocket. An album of photographs by his feet.

Lee went to see him and left a personal letter by his feet

He came home and I had a wake with his open coffin for all to see and say goodbye to. I played some of our favourite songs loud and didn't care that the neighbours would mind. I spent the night baking and went out and bought drink for the people that came.

Then we took him to the cemetery and placed him on a cold wet rainy afternoon into the ground on top of a hill onlooking the river where he used to love to fish. I picked up a handful of soil from the wet ground and threw it onto his coffin saying "Salt of the Earth!".

I asked the council if I could plant a tree which wasn't allowed. I planted expensive plants which later were stolen.

Whilst I was struggling to plant these plants on the stony hard ground of his grave my son was saying to me I shouldn't interfere with him and his girlfriend in Canada.

I had to interfere because he was living in a fantasy world with her and telling her things about himself that weren't true. I thought if she found out once he went to live over there with her she would end their relationship. I emailed her and she would not acknowledge his mental condition. So I told her. And she finished with him.

A week later I knew he was going to attempt his life. I stayed awake as long as possible but when I fell asleep for an hour I woke with a jolt and realised he had overdosed. Having abandonment issues that had never been addressed.

I desperately called an ambulance which took 40 minutes to arrive. I tried in vain to keep him awake. When the paramedics arrived they gave him a short of adrenalin.

Then drove him to intensive care. 40 miles away. I sat by his side as he was in a coma and knew there was nothing I could do so I went home by myself to a lonely house and couldn't come to terms with the way he did it and how he could do this to me.

I went back and he was semi conscious the next day. He couldn't move although they had him sat up because had contracted pneumonia again having had it once before when he was 5 years old. The nurses said because Lee was agitated fighting to regain the use of his body that they were going to give him medication. I mistook the medication to be a anti psychotic and was distressed because he had overdosed on them.

I emailed Ginger Breggin and she told me they were giving him a benzodiapine which was valium and I felt reassured. Nobody else was around to help me. I heard nothing from the mental health team at all.

As he regained consciousness he needed his glasses and I called Bro Hafren and my CPN took them to him. I couldn't face him. But eventually he came home and recovered then moved out into his own place which I am glad he has done.

In 2011 my next door neighbour's son harassed and then robbed me and went to prison for it. He was given a restraining order by the judge not to come near me or even onto my estate. Then in December 2011 I was admitted to hospital.

When I came out of hospital in January 2012 I started to experience harassment of a different kind. This time it was psychological. First of all I went to my local shop to buy food on a

Sunday and on the way back I could smell Sophie cooking a roast and said to myself well done her. Then the next morning there was a joint of meat on the path by my front door.

When I went out that week and wondered into a local shop which sold CD's on the shelf was a CD cover of the Dubliner's exactly the same as the one I had played Mark and beside it on the same shelf was a CD cover with the title Funeral something written on it. It shocked me.

The next thing that came over into my back garden was a carrot after I said to my son as he was leaving one day I was going to cook him carrot soup. Then my cat got hurt. One night I had an ex boyfriend call at my house and before he left I opened my back door to let my cat out and whilst the door was still open he said to me sometimes cats get run over and that night my cat got hurt. Someone had tried to grab him and hurt his belly I took him to the vets the next day and she said his front claws were pulled where he had gripped the ground and been dragged along.

Then I got tipsy because of this ex boyfriend and played a game with some small soft toys. I called by little soft toy kitten Anne junior and my little toy monkey Steve junior and sent pics of these toys to my ex boyfriend. Then I said out loud Anne junior has found another monkey and sent him picture of the kitten and another soft toy monkey kissing. The next day a banana appeared in my garden.

I was doing my gardening and got stung by a wasp and cursed out loud and then the next day part of a bees honeycomb nest appeared in my garden.

Then I took my garden tools to a neighbours house to help with her garden which was over grown and after a huge bramble appeared in my garden. I don't have brambles that size and it couldn't have blown over.

So I kept on calling the police who just laughed at me. And I started to read into everything that came into my garden. I thought my house was bugged or my laptop or mobiles had been hacked. I had a private investigator sweep my house for a listening device. I changed my lock and bought new mobiles and had my laptop checked. Nothing could be found.

Now I realise what happened. That my neighbours the Jacksons used to sit outside in their garden and with my windows opened and my back door opened they listened into my conversations. They saw me walk past their house through their kitchen window. And heard me tell my son I would cook him carrot soup when he was leaving my house and I shouted after him.

They did this to alarm me psychologically and it worked. They have given me no endless grief because of this. Simply for the reason I put Mark Jackson's son away in prison after robbing me. I never did anything to cause this family grief. I am just labelled mentally ill. And this to some people is enough. The Jackson boy is supposed to be a reformed character and told my son he was sorry for what he did to me. I forgive him. But I do not forgive his father for what he did to me. And the grief he has caused me over all of these years. I probably have a police record because every time I freaked out about something which came over into my garden coincidentally I called the police. I made accusations to police about who I thought was responsible not realising that I had been listened into by my neighbours the Jacksons. I have no evidence but I know it was them.

When I was in my garden and got stung by wasps I said out loud I wish that my other neighbours would do something about the wasps nest in their garden. And then part of a wasps nest appeared in my garden the next day. They heard what I said out loud over their fence.

They did this to torment me and it worked. I could never prove it to police and my CPN said I didn't know it was them all along. But then she wouldn't acknowledge my dystonia even though it was aggressive when I went up to see Dr. David Healy who wrote my GP about it. Saying it was caused by neuroleptics. I have a copy of his letter as proof. The police probably put it all down to my imagination because of what Kelle told them.

When Mark and I got married Maureen his sister was his witness at the registry office. At the time she was pregnant with her only daughter Tanya and she was born at the end of May 1978. We were married on the 18th May l978. Tanya grew up to be a beautiful blonde vivacious young woman but she had a fall from a horse and was in pain a great deal. The doctors couldn't find out what was wrong. She was prescribed pain killers and became addicted to them.

This led to further addictions then an addiction to heroin. At the age of 32 she died one week before Mark from an overdose of heroin. We buried them both on the same day and Mark never knew. She has left two young daughters behind.

Now it has been seven years since he passed. I live alone and actually love my freedom. I walk everywhere. I am learning Welsh. I go to the gym. I don't smoke any more. I work in my garden and it is a labour of love. I read and write a lot. And I paint. And I am learning how to play the drums. I have a good and active life. I am writing this book and have two blogs. One a poetry blog.

Mark and I were married for 33 years and I do not regret marrying him at all. I loved the man and will always miss him until the day I die. Mark was an honest and good living man. He was kind and intelligent with a wicked sense of humour. Most women said he was the perfect gentleman. He was not only my lover and carer he was my friend and confidant. We laughed and cried together. We lived and died. We went through hardship and good times. We travelled and played together. But when I think of Mark I remember his cheeky grin and most of all his laughter. This today echoes in my mind.

I am lucky to experience voices because sometimes one of those voices and the one I always want to be around me is his. He is telling me once again that he loves me. And I say back to him "I love you too". And I always will.

Chapter 12 LIVING

During February 2010 I had a very bad breakdown. I was withdrawing off my medication and my brain reacted and I became psychotic and delusional. My psychiatrist wasn't aware of and didn't know how to help me withdraw of my medication. It was his opinion I should remain on it for the duration of my life regardless of the side effects, which is brain damage and I was showing signs of it recently and wanted to avoid having it.

I even stripped off all my clothes only for lee to find me and call for help. Whilst I was ill that time I went out during the night at about 3am to buy tobacco from the all night garage. I came out of the store and there was a man in a car with two young teenage girls sitting on the back seat. I asked him if I gave him £10 would he drive me home to my estate and he agreed. The girls were giggling on the back seat of the car. The man was in his 30's or early 40's had dark wavy hair and was a little plump. He wore dark clothes. He took me home and watched as I opened my front door and went inside. Because I was so ill I forgot about it and was admitted but only spent two weeks in the hospital when I recovered well enough to go home. My doctor wanted me to stay for another three weeks because he was off on holiday. I said I wasn't prepared to do that. So on the condition I see another psychiatrist he let me go.

When I came home and lee left to move into a place of his own was when Elliot Jackson started to harass me aggressively by throwing things into my garden knocking on my door and generally being abusive when we met. In fact he started to harass me before when Mark came home to die. Then he robbed me. I was at the front of my house mowing the grass and I left my back door open when I finished and decided to go indoors. I was looking for something and noticed my purse was gone. So I realized Ellliot had taken it. I called the police and the officer found my purse in the shop refuse bin. Elliot also spent the money at the shop. It was as if he wanted to get caught and he did. In prisons they educate inmates on how to be rehabilitated. Elliot wanted to learn how to use a computer because he wanted to rake up trouble for the police on line. He has stopped now and his sister seems to have let up too. Except my Lee came up with the idea to befriend him on Facebook so we know exactly what he is up to.

I went to the station and gave a video interview to the police. Elliott Jackson was online praising the cold blooded murderer who shot down two young female police officers in a gangland killing in Manchester. And saying why didn't he come to Newtown to stamp out all of our pigs.

When I found out about this online I spilt a fresh cup of coffee all over myself and had to give myself first aid.

Then he was sentenced and locked up for one year. But I was put in hospital and lee had his elbow dislocated by a policeman and was in plaster for three months. We were both hospitalized. With fewer privileges than criminals.

I came home and that year Lee started to be more involved with some of the charitable societies and groups here. He had the patience of a saint teaching me how to use the computer properly. I started to write this book earnestly. But I was still grieving over Mark.

I had a drink and as usual fell into a deep sleep in my chair one night in my living room. I almost woke up because I felt there was a man dressed in dark clothes with dark wavy hair who was bending down over me and that he talked to me. I thought I must have dreamed it. But the thought also of someone breaking into my home got me really paranoid. I had my locks changed several times and lee's also.

I called the police out over and over believing someone was coming into my home whilst I was asleep. Things happened like my oven got mysteriously broke and fused my circuits when I used it so I was in the dark with no lights and just candles for three days.

I called 101 and the police at one time and these two police officers came and seemed to be making a social call. One of the officers came onto me and another asked for my phone number. The officer who came onto me wore a dark uniform had dark wavy hair and was plump. Just like the man who gave me a lift and the man I thought I had dreamed was bending down trying to talk to me whilst I was asleep.

It didn't occur to me at the time but they didn't have any radios. I complained straight away to the police and I have written to the complaints police department. The man broke in when I had a euro lock on my door which can be bumped with a bump key and the barrel not broken so you don't know is someone has been in. I have a wonderful relationship with Newtown Police. When I complained to the station about the two police men who treated their call out to me as a social call one officer on the telephone said their names were Robinson and Levington. I checked and there are no officers with those names working at my local station. Or at the station in Shrewsbury.

In October 2012 I was walking along the high street and crossed the road but the sun was in my eyes and I tripped on the curb and I fell full frontal onto the pavement. I dislocated my left elbow. I was taken to Shrewsbury by ambulance and was in plaster for 4 weeks. Lee did help a little but I was on my own with it. Coping with one arm and simple things like opening a tin of cat food by one hand and dressing yourself took a whole new way of strategy. Getting my bra on I really had to think about. So I fastened it and stepped into it and pulled it up over the plaster cast. Getting my socks on and dressed and washed took on a whole new way of doing. Everything from opening and closing my doors to doing my cooking and washing was difficult. But I was only in plaster for four weeks.

My cooker broke down and I have been using my microwave oven but I bought a new cooker for Xmas.

At the end of January 2013 I started on line dating. This was fun and safe but there is a sinister side to it and meeting up with someone to be alone with them is quite risky. The best website was Dating.mobi run by Andres Kellos. I had some real fun on their forum. But I also had a close call. A young man who was aged 27 came onto me and wanted me to stay in a hotel with him in Edinburgh. He said he would reimburse me with the bus fare. I was flat broke at the time and wasn't asking lee for £97 so I said he could pay by credit card and they would text me so I could prove my fare was paid for. He wouldn't so I told him to take his kilt and sporran and wrap them round his neck and strangle himself.

That was a close call because I didn't know this man or anything about him. He wanted me to stay in a hotel with him and was very handsome. He told me his dad was Jordanian and his mum Scottish. That he owned two car wash outlets. It ended and I finished it eventually.

I met up with Sexy Steve who came to see me but wouldn't pay for his own coffee let alone mine. This was terribly embarrassing. I was going to take the bill but a friend paid it for me and I didn't know who it was. I think it was my friend Angie? Steve said he was really broke and he had been unemployed for some time that he had come to Wales for a job interview.

After we had our coffees I showed Steve around Newtown. He asked me to hold his hand and I told him a little about myself and he told me about himself too. He said he was living with his mother and if it hadn't been for her he would have been homeless. That he was unemployed but owned properties and didn't want to sell them like the job centre said he had to and live off the equity. He wasn't given any benefits. But had a little rent from his houses that he owned.

He told me he played football two or three times a week for a local team in Wem where he lives. Recently he sent me some photos of himself and I think he is fit. I ran them off at the library and have them to keep. The first time we met which was approximately one year ago he asked if he could kiss me and I said yes so he kissed me twice.

He is online again tonight. Steve Jones and I have been chatting by text and email for months now and he is always saying he wants me and is coming onto me and tells me he will be with me soon but when I invite him over and he lives about an hours drive away from Newtown he says he is tied up. Just lately he dropped me the bombshell that he had a gorgeous girlfriend called Lynne and has been totally ignoring me not even telling me he didn't want to continue with me. I was pretty upset because I like Steve and I always will. Lynne lives in Walsall Birmingham way and Steve visits her every weekend. She has three children and is a 43 year old divorcee. He has been onto me again lately he wants sex or text sex because he can't have sex with his girlfriend. I told him I didn't want to bother with him any more. In fact I told him to fuck off! I feel so sorry for his girlfriend. He is always concerned about getting home at the right time. When he came I was under the impression he could only see Lynne every six weeks or so and was ready to have sex with him, but he told me he sees her every weekend only last weekend he was busy and they didn't have sex. He stroked my legs and said it would be our little secret. Then before I knew it he stripped off his clothes completely. He is nicely built for a 49 year old and I was sorry that he got dressed again but by that time I had already said I would not have sex with him.

In fact he bought me a cheap bunch of flowers and I threw them at him as he left and told him to fuck off. The next day there was something wrong with my cat Whiskas and I had to take him to the vets. The vet said he had been run over. Just before Steve left I let Whiskas out my back door and it was dark. Steve asked me if there was a main road at the back of my house because Whiskas could get run over. I thought this was rather a strange question to ask but didn't think anything of it. Then the next day the vet said Whiskas had been run over by a car.

I suspected Steve but I didn't know who was responsible and couldn't figure out why someone should do this. Or more importantly how had somebody overheard what Steve had said to me? I now know that my blackberry could also have given somebody access to my verbal conversations because somebody had hacked into it. I checked it out on line and it is possible and easier then people think. Steve never came across to me as malicious and when I confronted him about it he said he was an animal lover and would never hurt one. And I believe him. Somehow and I don't know how they overheard what he said to me. And this has been going on for years.

During the last eighteen months or so I have been hiring taxis from a company run by a wonderful lady called Debs. When Lee was really ill this last time he asked Debs to take him up to Cardiff to a music festival which was going on there. He paid her in advance and asked to be dropped off then picked up again a couple of days later. Debs went to find him but he was nowhere to be seen. Lee had left his mobile phone and all his stuff in her car and any other taxi driver might have sold it and pocketed the money. Debs couldn't access the phone and after asking the music festival organizers if they had seen anybody of Lee's description they hadn't.

I rang Lee's mobile from the Priory. Debs answered and explained. Then I got in touch with Bro Hafren and our local health team and also Cardiff police. Lee was eventually picked up and admitted to a psychiatric hospital in Cardiff. But they were talking of discharging him. Alan Davies our CPN from Newtown said he could go up to Cardiff and pick Lee up and bring him home but only on a Thursday and the hospital insisted that Lee had to wait and see a psychiatrist on the Friday. The psychiatrist said Lee should be discharged but by that time he had lost his credit card and had no money to travel the long journey back to Newtown. So in desperation I called Debs and asked her if she would go pick him up and I would settle up with her when I was discharged. So she got Lee back to Newtown safe and he was admitted to a hospital in Welshpool which is a town nearby us.

Debs is a very loveable, humorous and intelligent lady. She didn't say I was crazy when I told her just what I thought had been happening to me and the fact I thought I was being hacked on line, and being listened into. She is very knowledgeable about computers and mobile phones and told me it is quite easy to hack into a Blackberry, and other mobiles. I thought someone had been coming into my house to set this up which was extremely frightening for me and I had believed this all along. I was just told time and again by the police that nobody could enter my home. They can't now with bolts on my doors. And even if they enter whilst I am out they won't have access to my phone with me. I suspected my neighbours.

I met a really nice guy called Colin on line. Although he is not handsome and I don't fancy him sexually he came onto me and I did have on line sex with him for comfort reasons. Then when he said what he would like to do to me sexually I realized this relationship had to end too. He talked of putting a butt stop up my bottom and also putting his dick up there too. This Mark wanted from me years ago and as I am adventurous I tried it but it did nothing for me whatsoever and I found it rather uncomfortable. But most men want this.

But generally on the forums and talking to Americans was fun. My only competition on dating.mobi was Heikeva a very attractive

Swedish woman living in a small American town. She said someone travelled by greyhound bus half way across the States to see her then when he got there he tried to kill her. He is now in prison.

I learned from the Fraud Squad that African men put false identities on the website and that everything is false about them. They are after money. Most men are after on line sex which suits me as I don't want to live with anybody. And with text sex there is no physical contact. There is no chance of being raped or you catching an STD. And basically it is just masturbation with a little spark of delight from your on line lover. But the best way to find out if a man is a genuine guy is to check out his form. Someone who has plenty of interests, gifts, friends and who is on the forum regularly possibly is worth it. Also if there written English isn't very good then they are probably African. There are genuine people too and to discover these you check out their form. But be very careful giving out your address and meeting up with somebody who you are not sure of and always meet for the first time in a public place.

Lately there have been two African men coming onto me. One called blankey who asked me for money. And another young 23 year old coming onto me strong uses the name teesongz and I think his parents have put him up to trying it on with me so he can have a place in England to come over and continue his studies over here. These men are scammers and they should be reported on the scammers click on the dating site. Both these men asked for money.

For years taking psychiatric medications no psychiatrist or nurse had ever discussed sex with me and Mark and how these substances affect you sexually. Your sexuality. Impotency. Being obese changes the way you feel about yourself sexually for a woman anyhow and the drugs put stones on you in weight gain. No matter how hard I tried when I put myself on a diet it was like I was starving myself to death. And my weight never shifted. I never felt attractive. Now at this moment I am trying to on line date. To find sex. Not love or long term, because at the moment I feel nobody could replace my Mark, but sex. But if I met someone I could talk to and who would care maybe I would feel differently. I asked Dr Dhuma what about the weight gain he said to me you are responsible for anything you put into your mouth and have to watch what you eat. Then after that insult I said to him how difficult that was because he had such a wonderful chef at the Priory who baked a chocolate cake to just die for. And with nothing to do for hours a decent meal brakes the endless frustrating boredom but the food was incredibly stodgy. He didn't react well to my remark.

Mark couldn't gain an erection for 17 years. So that almost makes me some kind of virginal married woman. Not that he didn't try other ways but in this boring house he just couldn't break the boredom of it all either. He simply had no imagination.

I am seeing Dr Mohamad at 11am Friday. He wants to take me off all this cocktail Dr Dhuma has had me on. So I feel a little less threatened. But there will be no discussion or support with the horrendous withdrawals. I will call at the gym when my letter from the doctor is ready to get myself toned up.

One thing I do know coming off this cocktail Depakote, Clenazepam and Haloperidol has helped me a lot. Now I am just on 50mg injection of Haldol a fortnight which isn't much and I don't feel helps me at all. But at the moment I am sleeping. Which I do in my bed every night now. I called Paul Ashby the locksmith out again and this time had bolts put on both my back and front doors. This makes me feel more secure.

Chapter 13 ADMISSIONS

I have had two admissions to the Priory in Stockport this year. The first one I was discharged not well. But now after all Summer I am really well. In fact I have not been as well since before Mark died. But this is probably because of my circumstances that Elliot Jackson hardly harasses me and is no longer in the area and the man dressed in black no longer enters my house when I am asleep or not here.

Cheadle Royal Hospital The Priory was built in the 1800's and she is quite an old lady now. Sometimes you can smell sewerage. The showers overflow and flood your washing area. The washing machine is a circa 1952 antique. During this terribly hot summer no window could be opened. In fact there is perspex attached to each window which are mainly all authentic. To have new windows replaced would cost a fortune and The Priory is a private hospital now.

I told everybody that I was going to defend myself if they were going to force an injection on me. I was quiet and not kicking off when in the dining area they were ganging up getting ready to inject me. Unfortunately one of the nurses saying she was going to attend to another patient got in the firing line. I threw cold tea over her and stabbed her in the head with my felt tipped pen. This particular nurse had to stay off work for a few weeks because the wound got infected.

This sweet bubbly nurse turned out to be my favourite of all the nurses. She used to bring cakes and ice cream in for the patients bought with her own money. Nothing was too much trouble and was done for you with affection and humour. In a scuffle I pulled the ward managers hair and broke her glasses because I didn't want another injection.

I would kick off. When Dr. Dhumma told me I had to have the depot injection and I was outraged. I ripped the book An Unquiet Mind by Kay Jameison up to shreds which a young student nurse had loaned me and I stormed down the corridor reached a chair and flung it across the room like it was a cushion. But I never hurt anyone badly in all the years of being an in-patient. And these people did more harm to my mind and body with all the medication they were forcing me to take.

Being well and watching other patients kicking off I have seen how the staff handle them. They never shout but do raise their voices. The threat of an injection or the chill out room is always hanging over what they say and their authority. But there are special rules before the staff resort to keeping someone in the isolation room and there are always nurses present sometimes in groups holding

down that patient if they fight back. The whole system is specifically to break you and it achieves precisely this in almost every case.
Each nurse has an alarm and once triggered all the nurses run to help. They call this Response.
I have been against all the medication for years now but I thought that at one point that it worked. I was given haloperidol when the voices were strong. For two days of being medicated the voices moved from my shower room across to the other side of the room. Then they moved outside. A very beautiful young nurse told me that just above my shower room was a verandah where people sit and talk. She said not everything is inside your head Anne you know. That afternoon the voices had completely gone. Haloperidol might work temporarily or in my case just like a placebo. It was good nursing and the actual belief I had that it would work but it doesn't at all. And they are extremely toxic and dangerous to take. The withdrawals are bad too if not worse then the condition itself. I do not believe that they should be compulsory. I was a nuisance but I was not violently aggressive, although aggressive yes.
Dr. Breggin whilst being no charlatan works from his office and surgery. He also holds teaching sessions and gives talks and lectures on his expert knowledge of the harmful and dangerous affects of psychiatric medication. He has worked with patients in all criteria. The patients I saw all needed a place of sanctuary and although the NHS is suffering things are still nowhere near as bad as the amount of free care available in the States. Except it is possible to get justice and sue which is virtually impossible in this country against the NHS. Dr Breggin portrays bio psychiatrists as sell outs to the drug companies. That they don't understand their patients or the medication. In other words frauds. And I agree. They coerce you and blackmail you. They tell you they don't want you coming back but they know you will be and they hope you will because you are their bread and butter. No patients no doctors. In fact no psychiatric patients no psychiatric industry. No cleaners, electricians,carpenters, plumbers, office workers, secretaries, administrators, nurses, doctors etc. etc. No drug companies making billions from harmful toxins which are administered by doctor to unsuspecting and vulnerable people and children.
Sitting in the compound I tried to imagine Cheadle Royal as it used to be 200 years ago. It has always been a psychiatric hospital. The patients haven't changed the mad are still the same as they ever were. But the treatment for them has. Thanks to Dr Breggin pioneer that he is lobotomy has been stopped. Although I watched a documentary about OCD and how psychiatrists were drilling wires into people brains and placing a battery operated meter into their chests so that electrical impulses could be produced every time a

habit forming action was carried out. This failed to work and the patient could not stop crying.

Thinking of how Cheadle Royal was years ago I looked around in the compound.

There are still ten chimneys on the rooftops which meant three fireplaces going down on each floor from each chimney. Years ago the transport would have been horses and carriage. The gate keeper would have lived by the gate and the entrance and this door had long since been bricked up. The four large windows on the right of the compound would probably have been stables. There would have been no tarmac on the ground it would have all been cobble stones.

The nurses would have worn uniforms. Like I have said to people the mad have never changed but the treatments for them have.

All medication is compulsory. Everybody has to take it. I spent an hour with Dr Porter explaining why I did not want his medicine but he would not budge. They offered me a psychologist as talking therapy. She introduced me to ACTs Acceptance and Commitment Therapy. I read her book. She told me her mother had been diagnosed with schizophrenia and had made a complete recovery, was now in a high class job and living her life to the full. I never made a point of asking her how she had achieved this I only saw the psychologist once again at a ward round meeting although I was offered more sessions with her. I think I was frightened that although she said she had read Breggin all of my passionate beliefs would crumble and I wouldn't make it like her mother had anyway.

I had a conversation once with a senior nurse who had been nursing in psychiatry for a long time. I put the point to him that the mentally ill were only responsible for 2% of crime committed in 100% and I said why should the 99 percent of people be treated like criminals when they commit no crime for the sake of maybe one life. He said that he agreed to the 99% being locked up to save one life was more important and in any case most mentally ill were a nuisance. Why should people put up with the nuisance of us. That made me so angry and I let it show. I was imprisoned simply because I was a nuisance. In all medicine there is a risk. But doctors take that minimum risk for the majority of their patients. What this nurse said was totally unethical. But nevertheless it was his expert experience and only his point of view and not that of all of the nurses. He still helped me. When I was paranoid and delusional and up late one night. Although against the rules he succumbed and let me eat something and have a warm drink.

My key nurse wasn't much help. When he wasn't rushed off his feet he would spare the time to talk to me. He coerced me into thinking that the medication was going to help me. He also said that because I had been under so much stress and anxiety my nervous system couldn't take it any more so the least stressful thing that happened to me I would flare up and become extremely angry. And basically out of control completely. I said if they thought my nervous system was so fragile and anxiety inflamed it why was I placed in this high security hospital under lock and key surrounded by a high wire fence which would make anyone anxious. I laughed in his face at that prognosis. It was totally insulting to my intelligence and wellbeing.

They had the workmen in and with their noise and the constant slamming of the doors it was by no means a sanctuary, but I felt safe there because for the first time in years I wasn't having to live in fear of being alone in my home and someone coming in whilst I was asleep. Since my separation from Mark, his death and lee leaving and living alone.

The staff at Bro Hafren are stretched and poor in funds. Although Kelle Hall my CPN came out to see me and did some shopping for food for me and collected my prescription lately. I came off all of my medication. To prove to myself what was the symptoms of this and what was really me and not the illness. Also it was out of spite I suppose that I once again had been just dumped and left to do the real hard bit by myself alone. Knowing Kelle wouldn't do my shopping on a regular basis and I had to cope with housework and looking after myself after being carried about in hospital. I became kind of institutionalized. But I remembered what Mark had said that he thought Dr. Mohamad my psychiatrist was a good man. Mark was quite content to take the medication and was convinced it had helped him. In fact Mark was content to have his new car when he wanted and to eat good food and not have to work for it. Then when I split with him he had already come off all of his medication but I was told I still needed it and I thought to myself he is the one with a sound mind and well whereas I still get ill yet the responsibility for running the house and almost everything to do with our lives lay on my shoulders. And to me sex with Mark was a complete nightmare. In the end really he had given up. And was dragging me down with him. Although he said he still loved me the truth was he was dependant on me. And that was the difference.

I use the context and words "ill" and "well" because it is so ingrained in our society that to describe insanity it seems you have to say it is an illness but I don't believe it to be the case.

Everything on the Pankhurst ward we needed was catered for although it was under lock and key. Having everything done for you and the kitchen being locked and just a hatch to peer through was the ward policy also. But the nurses would make you a cup of tea or get you a snack any time. The food at mealtimes was tasty but fattening. And it was hard not to eat it and watch my figure. So I did put weight on. It was extremely stodgy. Sometimes the staff were too busy to make you a cup of tea and get you something to eat if they were run off their feet. But lunch and dinner were always catered for and a trolley was brought up from the kitchens.

This is what I remember about some of the women who were with me.

There was a woman who didn't talk sense at all. Everything was gobbledyguk. But she was like a child although she ripped the top off the pool table sometimes falling asleep underneath it. She would hallucinate and be in a world of her own. She turned all the arm chairs in the lounge upside down and they were heavy she pulled all the cushions out and made it impossible to sit in it. She would wear her clothes inappropriately. Sometimes putting gloves on her feet and knickers on her head. Or she would take her clothes off. The woman was a complete fascination to me because I had never come across anyone like her before. At first she grabbed my mobile out of my hand and I hung onto it for dear life. I was talking to lee. Then she noticed my bracelet and broke that. She knew more than what she was cracking on she did too. One night a huge group of nurses came to her room to inject her and she was like a wild animal. She had the strength of a gorilla. But the nurses seemed to hold affection for her and defended her against the women who complained to the nurses about her. I grew to love her. Once she was sat at the end of the corridor at the entrance and we both had huge pieces of cream cake, probably from somebody's birthday, in our hands. I became completely silly and encouraged this lady to have a pastry fight. We threw the cake onto the wall and I put some on my face. This might sound so ludicrous and insane but then is their different layers of sanity and I was already diagnosed insane anyhow. I did clear it up afterwards. It was just cake.

This lady broke my bracelet and the beads went everywhere but I found them on the floor where they had landed and picked them all up. The occupational therapist would come on the ward in the activity room and help us make bracelets from beads. I went to him and made a bracelet in tact out of the beads I had gathered up then I gave it to this woman who I knew was regressing and so ill. I grew to love her because she needed protecting. She was a woman in her late 30's and I was told she went into this insanity and regression then she would come out of it. She had the most beautiful face and hair and lacked inhibitions which she also needed protecting from. She needed dignity and the nurses did their best to give that to her. They knew how to look after her but never knew when she would lash out. Pulling hair or pulling things out of their hands like the observation folder. I grew to realize just how amazing her nursing care was at times but for whatever it was that had caused her insanity drugs were administered and probably if caught early with talking therapy and a different approach she would never have got so deep in madness.

Then there was a young lady who feared her new born baby would be taken from her. She had mental health issues and so did her partner and she didn't get along with the midwives and health nurses at the maternity hospital. I don't know all her background but it looked like she was about to lose her baby which was in foster care.

Then there was another lady who seemed rational one moment but was totally out of it the next. She lived on her own too and depended upon her ageing parents. We became friends then she turned on me. Accusing me of being Myra Hindley a woman who along with Ian Brady murdered several children in the 1960s. She was an extremely sick woman. Sometimes to those who didn't know her well she would appear quite rational, but in fact she was very ill.

Then there was a most beautiful young woman who had cut her wrists unable to leave her home. Agoraphobia ruled her life. She was congenial and sensible so she didn't stay too long and she was so glad to go home.

Whilst becoming myself I realized the actual role nurses play with their patients. At all times they are mostly polite and caring. They don't shout or lash out but they do place down boundaries. Then if a patient lashes out to another patient or a nurse they call Response and the patient is placed in the chill out room. Usually medication is used so 24 hour care is given and sometimes the nurses sit outside a patients bedroom giving care and observing their patient. They suffer verbal abuse nevertheless and occasionally physical abuse still they continue unhindered to give their patients the care they were trained to do.

Well, we will see what 2014 brings for us. New Years Day I took Lee for a meal to a 17th century hotel locally. We enjoyed it. But it is his birthday today and he doesn't feel good. He is down and feels groggy and sluggish in himself. My poor sweetheart does struggle at times. Hope I can see him soon to give him my gifts and cake and card. Its such a shame to watch him like this as he struggles. I took him for an Italian meal recently, which we both enjoyed. He really helps me and I hope I help him too. He has his charity work that he does and he belongs to a peer group which gives him support.

I took myself off to the pub again last Saturday night and did get some attention. It wasn't a bad night out and I met some lovely young people. I met this Lord somebody who bought me a drink but disappeared when I told him my age which is 62 now. I find this terribly amusing. People say I look about in my mid fifties.

It was a friend who pointed out to me that I was an activist for a while when I was in my early twenties. I went on marches with feminist women. I read Spare Rib and the Female Eeunoch . And even though I have never been close to another feminist I would love to be
I am aware of the young Sean Rigg who the police murdered.
I am determined irrevocably to finish this book.
 I am lonely but I have my interests. I have a life. I cannot say I will never go insane again but I feel very confident that I won't. I have the psychiatrist off my back and I do not suffer from extreme withdrawals any more because I take a small amount of the Haldol injection.

Chapter 14 SMOKING

I always smoked around Mark and it was one of the first things he did getting me hooked on smoking. I was on a dipixol injection at Xmas time 1977 and this had a terrible affect on me. It made me feel really low and depressed. I was staying with Mark and his mum and Mark kept on offering me cigarettes. Although I didn't smoke when pregnant with my Lee and not properly until Lee was around 5 years old. Lee has never smoked. Now I have quit for 4 years.

I titled this book Virginia Art because smoking played a big part in my life whilst I was married to Mark. We always smoked the tobacco Golden Virginia. So I took Virginia from that. Then years ago Mark read Lord of the Rings by Tolkein three times. When we went to watch the films in one caption Frodo Baggins is smoking his pipe in the Shire with Sam and they call smoking the Art. So I decided to take the Art from there. Virginia Art.

Smoking has been around in Britain since the 15th century when Columbus first brought the tobacco plant back from the Americas.

It started off that both men and women smoked then it became a strictly male ritual. Then women who thought of themselves as liberated smoked in public and during the 1950s when the movies and films influenced people and became incredibly popular advertising and film stars made it popular for both sexes. They made it appear sensual and glamorous. And as cigarettes were cheap it became popular among the classes and trendy. Mark was caught up in this as was his dad but the women of his family didn't smoke. It was a manly thing for him to do. Part of growing up.

Now of course it is considered a health risk to smoke and I really feel better not smoking any more myself. I never liked the addiction. Smoking broke my marriage up. Mark smoking destroyed our relationship. Mark was a spiritual man. He believed if he had faith in Jesus he would live forever. It was that simple for him. Just believe in Jesus and God and you will live forever. I believe he is still around me and he always will be. Little things that just can't be explained could be Mark making his presence known to me.

Dr. R. D. Laing wrote a chapter heading in his book The Politics of Experience that goes like this:

Jesus said to them:
When you make the two one, and
and when you make the inner as the outer
and the outer as the inner and the above
as the below, and when
you make the male and the female into a single one,
so that the male will not be male and

the female not be male, when you make
eyes in the place of an eye, and a hand
in the place of a hand, and foot in the place
of a foot, and an image in the place of an image,
then you shall enter the kingdom.
(the Gospel according to Thomas)
I do not believe Jesus was the son of God. I do not believe in God.
This is a patriarchy thing. The equivalent of the supreme male
being and the son thereafter. We have had patriarchy for
thousands of years but 2,000 years ago this world was dominated
by Amazons. There was no such thing as male dominance over
this planet and its beings. I have read such wonderful women such
as Mary Daly, and her wonderful books Gyn/Ecology, Pure Lust
and Outercourse. Simone de Beauvoir, and her book The Second
Sex and Bell Hooks, Luce Irigaray and of course Germain Greer
and her books the Female Eunoch and The Climacteric. I have
read about women writers like Olive Schreiner, Gertrude Stein,
Anais Nin and strong women like Mae West, Margaret Mitchell,
Zora Neale Hurston and Doris Lessing to name just a few. And
women with a rich tapestry of life like the beautiful Katherine
Hepburn.
I log onto blogs such as Feminista, RadFem and the F Word. And I
keep an eye on feminists in America.
I am a feminist before I am a mother, daughter, sister or aunt. And
always will be. I believe in it passionately and always will until I die.

Now 5 years after Mark has died I feel my own person again. I get
along with everybody well and I am confident. I know Mark is
around and feel his presence and I know he is forgiven and wants
me to be happy. I am not looking but a male friend would be nice
and I find that at my age of 63 I am having more passes and
attention from the opposite sex then I was when I was in my 40's
and 50's. Which is nice.

I live for Lee my son he still needs me having his own emotional
problems and being in hospital at present. I will see him right.

Recently my father passed away at the fine age of 92. He left some
money to us three and I have never had so much in all my life. It
was £10,000. I am having a new bathroom put in and a walk in
shower because I fell in my bath and the workmen are doing a
really wonderful job for me.
I like living here in Newtown it is home and the weather has been
wonderful lately. Glancing at the surrounding hills of this Welsh
valley makes me feel uplifted just as it always has.

I am aware of some of the history of Newtown. Robert Owen is the man most known in its history. The person who interests me most in Newtown's history is Emily Briscoe. She was a wealthy landowner here in Newtown and lived in the house which is now the current Town Hall.

For Queen Victoria's jubilee the town councillors were deciding on what to build in the town as a commemoration to celebrate. They raised £500 and couldn't decide on how to best use it. There was talk of building a bridge, a tower and creating a library and the councillors wanted all three which meant they would still be paying for all of this even today. So Emily stepped in. She owned the buildings and land at the Cross in Newtowns town centre. She also owned other land on Park Street.

She put the proposal to the councillors that if she pulled down buildings on the Cross she would build one amazing structure and clock tower. She would also build a library on condition the councillors joined the new lending books law and also if they gave her the £500. The councillors were of the opinion that common people wouldn't be interested in a library because they were all illiterate and therefore it would be of no use. But children were being taught how to read in school and it was bound to be a success.

So the councillors agreed and the building of the clock tower went ahead. The library was also built. The wonderful building is still standing and the clock still gives accurate time. The current library is a new one because the old one burnt down in the1980's. But it is much appreciated and has been invaluable over the years for many people to enjoy me included.

So Emily left her mark and not many people know about her and what a remarkable lady she was.

I consult my therapist who is absolutely wonderful. Mick and I have become friends although we have never met and he is there for me all the time. I consult him by phone. I have never had talking therapy before and know if Mick had been around for me when I first started with the symptoms of madness aged 16 I would have been helped immensely and probably would have made a complete recovery eventually.

I still break down and end up in hospital and recently was admitted again.

I feel well at present. Apart from the odd aches and pains I am healthy and soon my medication will be reduced once again. Although the Haldol affects me and embarrassingly my chin has been wobbling. This is like a symptom of Parkinsons Disease. To counteract this I chew gum and somehow this stops it.

Thanks to dad and his inheritance I can have a new bathroom built in which is going on at the moment.

Also I am looking to lose some weight which the medication has put on me and I will be going back to the gym.

I am positive about the future. I feel I might live to a ripe old age and hopefully keep my health.

At Dad's funeral I met my brother and sister again. Also my cousin Terry. It was wonderful to be reunited with them all. I also met Chris's eldest boy who looks the spitting image of Cashek. Which was wonderful.

Dad going is the end of an era. Whilst in the Priory last year I thought I saw David's ghost. I was texting my brother who was at my Dad's bedside whilst he was dying. I said to Chris didn't David die in April just at that time of year and that I thought I had seen his ghost. Then Chris told me Dad had just passed away that very moment. I don't know if that did actually happen or Chris made me believe it did and lied about it simply because he wants me to believe in an after life?

Recently the Jacksons have left and moved on. And I have new neighbours who are lovely.

After having another admittance this year and Lee becoming quite bad and being admitted too I started having my jaw moving irregularly and this is one of the first signs of brain damage. So what is happening with me now is that they have reduced my Haldol injection. They are doing it quickly and I find I am suffering withdrawals.

But I have been consulting my therapist Mick Bramham and he has been a wonderful support. I have been able to afford him with my inheritance and he is there when I text.

For the past couple of nights I haven't slept well and this morning I woke up with a nightmare about my son. But my therapist has advised me what to do and is a great comfort. He has actually met Dr. Breggin once in America and I have absolute faith in him.

Mark believed in the doctors. His mother brought him up that way. He believed in the medical and psychiatric doctors and nurses. When I was in hospital as an in patient with him years ago I used to watch him form relationships with the psychiatric nurses. I saw it as collaborating with the enemy. When as an out patient he visited the psychiatrist they used to talk but never discuss our financial situation and the fact we weren't allocated the money we should have been getting.

His one and only friend was a man who drank and smoked pot and he died a few years before Mark. I wondered just what I had married even though deep down I think I still loved him. But I hated our lifestyle and I had my wonderful son to live for. He needed me more then ever.

During January 2012 when I left hospital to come home after my neighbour's son robbed me and harassed me the family started to harass me in a different way. They would listen in to my conversations at my front door when I was stood there. And listen in when they were sat in their back garden to my conversations through my open living room window and back door.

When my son came home from hospital I told him at my front door as he was leaving that I would cook him some carrot soup the following Sunday when he came to dinner. The day after a carrot appeared on my back garden path. There is a just a field at the back of my house and no people pass by there. My next door neighbours had put it there. Just to harass me. Then when I stung myself on a wasps nest in my garden they had been next door in their garden and heard me and the next day they put part of an old bees nest in my back garden. They probably had one in their garden. Never doing any gardening much and their grass always being over grown.

Then when I had the affair with Steve Jones and he told me he had a girlfriend he was seeing every week yet he came to me for sex a few days after he left I got drunk a little and took my soft toy a monkey I called Steve Junior and another soft toy I called Anne Junior which was a kitten and put them together making love and kissing and I text him with these images. Then I trashed Steve Junior in the bin and text him with these images. Then I got another soft toy another monkey and put the kitten soft toy together with it kissing and said out loud to myself "Anne Junior has found another monkey to love!". I had my window opened and one of the Jacksons must have overheard whilst sat outside smoking in their back garden next to mine and a couple of days later a banana appeared on my back path. Which although amusing became distressing for me because it was happening all the time.

Then I went to see and help out an old lady a couple of blocks from where I live. I cut myself on her brambles. I went back but she had been sent to a home because she was suffering from dementia. I passed by the window of my neighbour's house carrying my garden tools. When I came back I had left my tools at the old ladies house but was looking at my bramble cuts on my arms as I passed my neighbours kitchen window. Then they put a huge bramble in my front garden. I kept calling the police and they wouldn't do anything. I kept reading into everything that was thrown in my garden. All the rubbish had some sort of meaning to my life. Like if I was in the taxi talking to my friends Debbie and Jayne a taxi wrapper would appear in my garden and I would wonder who put it there. For years I read into everything coming into my garden and it gave me untold misery and fear. I wondered who was doing this to me and why? I told the police and they laughed at me.

Then this year 2015 I had a CCTV camera fitted in the front of my house covering my garden. And I suspected something had been thrown over. I called my security engineer out to see if he could help. Then he noticed the piece of paper I thought had relevance and he told me it appeared on the screen before I decided on what I was going to do and it couldn't have any relevance. So I realised I had been reading into everything since 2013 and the bramble appearing in my garden.

I have a five star cylinder lock on my door and a bump free lock on my back door. My windows are locked with a key. And I have dead bolts on both my doors. I am as secure as I would be if I was living in Fort Knox.

I decided to title this book Virginia Art and took the word Virginia from the Golden Virginia tobacco we always smoked it being the cheapest and most enjoyable taste. And I took the word Art from Lord of the Rings and Frodo Baggin's moments he spent with Sam in the Shire where they sat smoking their pipes calling it The Art. So Virginia Art.

Chapter 15 LIVING

I was browsing the net recently and found out about a conference being held in London at the Roehampton University. It was a conference headed Psychiatric Medications More Harm then Good. So I decided to go. My little cat Whiskas who had had liver desease these last three years finally lost his fight and died. So I was free with no ties. I couldn't get a ticket at first then I applied as a delegate and bought a more expensive ticket a day before the deadline. I booked a room in a nice little hotel for two nights and bought a ticket for the coach which was a direct route to London.

When I arrived in London I settled in my room then went for a lovely meal at a Moroccan restaurant. The next morning I showered and had an English breakfast early at a local cafe on King Street. Then I took a taxi to the University. The taxi driver found the part of the university it was to be held in.

I was one of the first to arrive and met Jasmine and Anne. Two women who have physically disabled sons. Anne had a disabled child because she was prescribed psychiatric medication when she was pregnant. Jasmine had a son who had a bike crash and then was prescribed medication and suffered from it as well as being in a wheelchair.

I met the wonderful Sandra Breakspear. She told me she is attempting to set up a clinic which sounds amazing. Called Chy Sawel in St. Ives. Her son totally being damaged by neuroleptics and incarcerated these past ten years. She said she would never give up fighting for her son.

I talked to others and had my say. I interrupted Peter Gotzsach. Why? Not because I didn't admire the man for what he was saying but because what he said hurt so much. He mentioned sexual issues caused by these drugs. My Mark had erectile dysfunction when we first slept together. And for the last 17 years of his life. What Peter Gotzsach said hit a nerve and hurt beyond words. I myself have not been effected but Mark was most of his life.

I met the wonderful Dr. Peter Breggin by Skype who could not attend in person because his wife had a small stroke and he wanted to be with her. I asked him questions about Parkinson's of which I think I might be suffering because I have been having dystonia. He said everyone is so different and I might not have it at all or that bad. I am reading a book by Oliver Sacks who died on the same day as my cat.

I also met the amazing journalist Robert Whitaker whose books I have read and am reading one of his books at the moment. He wrote Mad in America and Anatomy of an Epidemic. I am reading his book The Mapmaker's Wife which is about an expedition of men who took place in the 17th century who discovered the world was round and a woman who trekked the Amazon in search of her husband. I haven't quite finished it yet. But am enthralled. It is steeped in history and is a remarkable tale it would make a wonderful film and I believe one director is looking to do this with it.

I heard of the Open Dialogue Treatment in Lapland Finland which I already knew about and how people there were getting an 86% recovery rate for first time experience of psychosis. This is family therapy done in the home. I found out about a conference for this next February 2016 in London and have already bought a ticket and intend to go. I would simply love to train in this but they only train professionals which I am not so doubt if I would meet their criteria.
This is the way forward for people with psychological overwhelm at any time in their lives. This deals with the person as a whole unit not detached. Treatment involves family and friends or anybody connected with a person who has ties and knows them. And mostly who love them.

I intend to become active and I want to be an activist on mental health issues. Especially against drug inducement and incarceration. I would like to see a change in the law. I am aware of the voluntary organization PAVO and hope to attend their seminar. Which is local.

Mark would be proud of me. And I feel this is the way forward for me and my son and it will somehow give him hope if he sees what I am doing.

And as the old saying goes "Where there is life. There is hope!"

I am amazed to still find myself alive today. After so many attempts on my life that failed and i now realize I was meant to stay alive. I was meant to stay alive for my son.

Like the three devoted mothers who I met recently at the conference in London I want my son to be happy foremost in my life. It is part and parcel of my own happiness.

Adam Faith was a singer and actor in the 1960's swinging era of the UK. Before he died he was asked the question who had inspired him most in his life. Adam said that the person who inspired him the most was the founder of the food chain empire MacDonalds. When they met Adam asked him what was his philosophy on his success. This person replied. "You don't need money to be successful. You don't need education. All that you need is determination!"

I have been determined to write my story and this book. To somehow make a very small difference to the lives of people who suffer from psychological overwhelm.

But mainly I have written this book to prove to my son that he can one day find happiness in his life. Happiness cures all human ails. Also in the animal kingdom this goes without saying. A happy animal is a great thing to behold.

Happy human beings achieve the most remarkable things on Earth.

Happiness has always been the goal of everyone. Happiness is worth more than all the gold in the world. I am happy to have had the opportunity to write this book thanks to my wonderful son who has taught me with the patience of Job how to become computer literate.

And the story is not over.

Chapter 16 SANDRA'S STORY

This is the story of Sandra Breakspear and her son Anthony. Who already I so admire and feel affection for although we have only just met.

Sandra came up to me as I was sat on a bench just after lunch at the London conference More Harm Than Good psychiatric medications which was held on 18th September 2015. And can be found on YouTube. I spoke out.

I was immediately struck when she told her story at least part of it. She mentioned her project Chy Sawel and her son Anthony who has been detained under Section in a mental institution these past ten or so years.

Knowing about the distances people are sent I asked how she managed to visit her son. She said one visit took her 6 hours there to him and 6 hours back. And she did it in one day. She explained how he is constantly psychotic and paranoid and when she goes to give him a hug he moves away. Which would break the heart of any ordinary mother and break her spirit too. Not Sandra. This has made her even more determined to fight for this child of hers who she raised and gave birth to. Who she will always treasure and love.

Her project could help save my son and her cause is now my cause. I will do everything in my power to help her.

I feel that my son has been damaged by psychiatric medications but that this with the right treatment could be reversible. Chy Sawel would give the right treatment to my son. The right support. The right way to recovery. And a life changing approach to his every day existence.

Sandra told me a little about herself. That she was struggling to raise funds. She was nursing her 81 year husband who had just had two major strokes, getting very little support and had just been caring for her two great grandchildren whilst her daughter had been away.

Sandra said her parents were from Jersey and during the war were occupied by the Germans. Her mum and dad were sent to Germany.

To me she is a most amazing person. To have fought for so long the long uphill fight to save her son and get him out of the psychiatric institution where he is drugged with damaging intoxicating medicines which breaks her heart but not her spirit every time she visits him.

This woman has been determined. I am determined. Together we will win this fight for our sons sake.

Tomorrow I am going to try and speak to Dr. Astrid Bonfield a National Lottery board member. To literally put this cause to her and obtained lottery funding for Sandra and her dream.

Somehow I will raise the money for Sandra. Somehow!

Then as I looked into all of this attempting to help Sandra Mick said to me you are looking into two different projects and I realised I was. I was looking into my own project.

They have had success in Sweden with the mentally ill living on farms. This gave me an idea and I came across a farm house down in Cornwall. Then I thought well there are farm houses here where I live in Newtown. And I have taken it from there.

I want to start a project of my own. I want to buy a farm house and small holding. To rent out the rooms to young teenagers who are just suffering psychosis for the first time. And hire a psychiatrist, psychotherapist, nurses and occupational therapist and treat these young girls. I would have animals on the small holding, donkeys, chickens, cats, dogs and a cow from which we would make cheese and cream, and the girls would be involved with their up keep. I would start with girls then boys because I know girls being a woman myself.

And I would grow vegetables and have a small orchard. And they would be involved with this. And also they would have art, music, yoga and writing therapy. They would cycle in the countryside and fish. And get involved with the local college and recreational facilities learning coping and social skills.

They would be treated by the open dialogue therapy which involved families. Which has an 86% success rate in Lapland,Finland. They would not be prescribed medication or forced to do anything they didn't want to do.

There was a William and Mrs Ellis in the 18th century who had a similar house and they had such success and were admired by a famous journalist at that time in an article she wrote.

I have spent the last week night and day looking into it. I have the approval of Bob Whitaker. And our friend Marion Aslan award winning nurse who works training nurses in the Elemental nursing procedure and with the Thrive care plan. She wanted my son to work for her promoting this but unfortunately he has not had the confidence never wanting to venture from his home town.

I got in touch with Nick Putten at the training centre for open dialogue therapy in London and he approves.

Also Millie Kieve the charity worker for APRIL.org also thought it was a good idea.

And Jason Pegler the publisher who runs chipmunkapublishing.co.uk who will publish this book for me was very helpful with ideas.

I am trying to attract an investor and raise funds.

This is another dream. But a dream I wish to make reality. A dream I wish to make come true. I would call the house David's House. After our brother David who committed suicide by hanging after he asked me about medication and I said I didn't think it worked. He had no hope but believed in Jesus and went to join him in heaven. He would have been 61 years old last August and he was 22 years old the day he died in the April of 1976 and my father aged 92 passed away in April 2015.

Alas for me this is only a dream and a dream I know probably will never come true.

Chapter 17   MY SON

The love of my life was Mark but the one person who has inspired me for the last 36 years and almost as long as I have been involved with psychiatry is my son Lee.

He was born in the cottage hospital in Newtown on Monday the 8th January 1980 at 8.45am. I had a very healthy pregnancy free from medication and riding my bike around our sleepy town having fresh air and a really nourishing diet.

Before he was born and heavily pregnant I would ride everywhere on my bicycle and towards the end I could feel a little hand wanting to come into the world from beneath me. Then after watching the last episode of a series of Blake 7 on TV with Mark on a Sunday night I started in labour. Mark phoned his aunty and she drove us to the hospital which is situated on a high hill at the top of our town.

Mark missed the final episode of Blake's 7 which he had been following because I was told to walk around and I became quite frightened at the daunting prospect of what lay ahead of me. And as it was my first child I didn't quite know just what to expect. I knew it would hurt like hell.

Wanting to do what the midwife Sister Jones told me her saying she had lambed many a sheep and that they were creatures who gave up on life easily unlike human babies. But I remember in the middle of winter being out on the grounds of Telgarth in Brecon and in the snow walking and seeing a little lamb trying to shelter with its mother against the harsh wind and snow along a fence. To me Sister Jones had it all wrong and that all babies need nurturing and care especially if they are out in the cold and mum is trying hard to protect them.

I always tried and attempted to protect my son who was a beautiful baby and a gorgeous child and is a kind and loving insightful intelligent handsome man.

For the first six months of his life I breast fed and nurtured him and was in the process of weaning him with Johnson's baby food in jars amongst some small amount of the food I prepared for us. Then Mark put in for voluntary redundancy from the factory where he earned good money. Maggie Thatcher became prime minister and the black recession came to Newtown where factories which employed many closed down. Industry went bleak. And shops also packed up and left and the high street was also bleak. But we were settled although I realised it meant being back on benefits for a long time. I had the offer from Mark's mum to go back to Manchester but our house on the estate where we have always lived was a nice house with a back garden and the alternative was living in a council house in Manchester where already Mum's neighbours Aunty Alice and Uncle Joe had been robbed three times.

Many might not have agreed with the policies of Margaret Thatcher but I think it was her misfortune that a global recession came about just as she was elected into power and I think the woman has gone down in history as a very skilful and talented prime minister who had the gumption to bring into her cabinet John Major whose government introduced Disability Living Allowance which brought millions out of poverty my family included. Although I now know I have lost so much losing my nursing and secretarial careers because of the stigma bio psychiatrists and psychiatric workers do nothing but increase.

Mum and dad were struggling and had been turfed out of their flat where on the landings were found syringes from druggies who had sheltered there from the cold night. My parents had been allocated an awful cold and meagre place because Manchester City Council were modernising their flat and they had to huddle around a little gas fire to keep warm.

So I decided to stay put because like Mark often told me the crime rate at the time in Newtown was minimal and we had Mum's sister Aunty Mary who was some support. Back then you could leave your back door unlocked which I know I can still do but my house is extra safe now. I placed bolts on my front and back door and set up a CCTV camera at the front.

This I did because I needed protection with what had happened to me over the years as I had been a victim of crime after Mark died in 2009.

When Mark finished at the factory because it was closing down Lee was just a baby and I went totally into emotional overwhelm and became delusional through lack of sleep and my imagination running wild at what disasters lay ahead of us all.

I became paranoid and had hallucinations. So my mum was called up and came to stay but I tried to escape through a downstairs window away from Mark because I thought that both of them were going to kill me and sell my baby to some other family. This I know that when a person becomes emotionally overwhelmed if they have been prescribed psychiatric medication in the past the chemical imbalance is still there and remains. Once delusional and psychotic sometimes it never goes away and the brain being what it is brings it back. But after talking therapy I don't get as emotionally distressed any more. I don't feel guilt or shame. Mark in some respects made me feel this and I don't feel it any more.

There was a struggle when I tried to get through the window with Mark holding onto me because he was trying to stop me running away and he had to protect me somehow from myself. An ambulance was called and two paramedics in uniform came around to the back of the house and grabbed me and I was dragged away screaming out they were going to kill me. I was taken 50 miles away to Telgarth in Brecon. Beforehand all the neighbours came outside and the gossip started about me and how crazy I was and they felt sorry for my poor baby who was just six months old.

Mark had a new baby on his hands and was worried what to do so he took out our bank savings and bought a little car on hire purchase then he brought me from Telgarth and drove his mum, Lee and me and took us to the mother and baby unit back at Withington in Manchester.

Dad being who he was didn't weigh up the situation and decided he would ask Mark to drive my two cousins who were on holiday over from Poland back to Wales so they could see something of the UK.

Then my mum and dad came up and they all had to come back home and there was no room for all four of them in the small Datsun and Mark sensible as he was said he wouldn't drive mum and dad home and they had to find their own way back and they had another massive argument. Mark hadn't slept properly for days and on his way back from returning my cousins took a wrong turning because his eye was sore and he couldn't focus properly or see and he ended up in Wrexham in the middle of the night swerving and driving badly. The police tracked him down and revoked his licence and he was shipped of to North Wales to a hospital where he said at Denbeigh he was placed on wards with the criminally insane.

His brother and wife visited him and took a watch Mark had traded and gave it to the nurses who pocketed it. And Anne went to the ladies and got locked in terrified she wouldn't be let out.

During my stay on the mother and baby unit I continued to feed Lee Robinson's baby food which came in a dried food little box you mixed with boiling water. Mark's mum travelled to Altrincham from Northenden in Manchester every other day and brought it to me. Otherwise Lee would have been taken from me and placed into care because when I was told by a nurse that the canteen would make up some baby food for me all the other babies being newly born when they brought it to me it turned out to be fish gruel with all the bones still in it.

The nurses were told I had to feed and change Lee and wash his clothes which I carried on doing. I saw a psychiatrist once and I told him about some of the delusions I was then having. One was I thought the sounds of overhead aeroplanes were Mark's brother riding a motorbike on the roof trying to get passed the security of the hospital to kill me. I imagined I had been shot once when mistakenly listening to the dryer in the laundry room. All figments of an over active imagination then as always.

So Lee was moved to the nursery so I could lie in and get some rest but the nurses left him to cry and his cries reached me so I got up anyway to feed and play with him. Teaching him through his first walking steps and giving him the toys there to play with.

So like my son has just said to me he has spent 35 years of his life in institutions and on medication. Having being separated from us as early as three when he was taken out of the orphanage by Mark's sister Mo and taken to stay with her and her family of three boys and Tanya her only girl. Every time Mark and I were sent into hospital together Lee went to family. Mark made sure he was safe and out of care and we never lost him to social services.

So the years went by. And Lee found the neighbourhood kids used to bully him having one young boy coming to play with him and sticking up for him who he ran to for protection. He too is a young man now and is a little older then my Lee but he has the muscle wasting disease muscular dystrophy and soon will be wheelchair bound. I still bump into his mother on the bus and she is a lovely Welsh lady. She is a friend.

Lee went to Cornwall when he was 8 years old and spent his birthday with Mark's brother his wife and boy Gary. They lived in a flat at the time which was over a butchers shop.

From the age of 3 onwards Lee had issues and I was asked by the school nurse just what I was intending to do about his disruptive behaviour. The same woman was the mother of the older boy who bullied my Lee and hit him across the back of his legs with an old pram frame once. I was constantly going round to her house to tell her to keep her son away from mine.

When Lee was almost three years old in December 1982 and his mummy was taken away his dad brought him to see me at Telgarth and my further admittance once again. Not before Mark was angry with the situation and when walking the return journey down the path from the town centre to our home with Lee he wouldn't wait for him and his little steps. Before then Mark used to carry him upon his shoulders and he was so upset he took it out on little Lee. Then he was ill himself and Lee was placed in the local orphanage where very reluctantly they gave him over to Maureen who came to get him out of there.

Lee when he was 3 years old and separated from me for the first time was brought with Mark to Talgarth where I was and he wouldn't talk to me at all and was already traumatized. But there was no way I was consulting a child psychiatrist and having his welfare and well being brought into the hands of doctors who believed in drugs and shock. There was no way I was involving him with a child psychiatrist then although he has always been wrapped up in the psychiatric system. My heart will always be broken because of this and I pray some day he will be free.

My mission was to protect my son and that has always been my total priority being too ill at times to know what to do for the best and making mistakes along the way but otherwise giving him much love and quality time.

Mo and Arthur that December in 1982 went bankrupt and lost all their possessions and their home. Mo went off the handle and had an affair and Arthur hit her one night when we had arrived to collect Lee after both being discharged from hospital and set free once again. Tanya was traumatized and crying and Mark was so drugged he didn't wake up. I was told that Mo had this affair and Arthur had hit her. I wasn't told about their bankruptcy and they were heading for homelessness. They later rented a cottage in their village and got allocated a council house later on. Now they are retired and living in Spain and I thank Mo for everything she has done. She is the kindest sweetest woman I know although she is as fierce as a tiger mother with her cubs.

We were poor then and I had no good winter coat. And whilst in hospital I had to break it to Mark that Mum Watmough had passed away that December. Xmas is a bad time and I wanted to cancel Xmas so much this last year and I had a go at my Lee who was already showing signs of overwhelm. Having come off his medication too quickly but not hearing any the advice from me just what can happen when you do.

I got angry with him because he questions my judgement and really doesn't accept that sometimes. Just sometimes. Mum knows best!

Then for all of his life there have been times when he has witnessed me becoming totally out of character irrational and my behaviour has become absurd. So he tends sometimes to doubt my judgement.

He has been embroiled in the psychiatric system all of his life. He had his 36th birthday last Friday on the 8th January 2016. Now he is incarcerated in the Priory, Cheadle Royal Hospital, in Cheshire.

He has been admitted many times. It all started when he was suffering from severe anxiety and depression because his issues had never been addressed. He had issues with abandonment and trauma stemming from his childhood since the age of three.

I tried a therapist with him that our Mental Health disapproved of and he responded to this but she was limited in what she was capable of and experienced in. She was fully qualified and trained just not in the right methods and in ways she could help my Lee work through his issues.

My therapist is a fully qualified psychotherapist with many years experience and he has been absolutely wonderful for me. I tried encouraging my son to consult him but like all children and he is now a man he had to find his own way. And doubted my judgement anyhow.

My therapists name is Mick Bramham and he has a website Myths & Risks and also a blog. I found him on Mary Maddocks Mind Freedom in the USA from David Oaks website and his blog touched my heart when he wrote all about his grief from his lost dog Boris the beautiful Border Colley he adored.

Mick has many years experience attending boarding school when a child and having two grandmothers who had mental health issues. His brother is a famous artist. He lives down in Weymouth Dorset and we have never met but I consult him by Skype, email, text and by phone. And he sent me flowers once when I had an admittance.

He started his career working in a residential home for disturbed young boys where the psychiatrist who ran it did not believe in drugging the children in his care.

Then Mick went on to run a charity which helped the mentally ill also, which after led him on to train as an existential psychotherapist.

I owe him so much. I owe him for my sanity! I know God has worked through him and cured me now.

My son was allocated another therapist outside the Mental Health Team and this he says really helped him work through his issues of depression.

When I first was informed through reading a book titled Toxic Psychiatry by Dr. Peter Breggin a psychiatrist who works in New York with his wife Ginger, I had the dilemma of knowing my husband was on medication and remaining well. In fact he had remained well and without any signs of mania for 17 years.

My opinion is that these medications only work when the Placebo effect is in motion in a person's mind. They do not have any chemical qualities which aid emotional overwhelm which is always due to experiences of trauma.

When my son was first starting to become overwhelmed I was desperate like most family members and parents. I looked at my husband and had the only glimmer of hope available medication. So we referred him to our GP. Who overdosed him, started an adverse chemical reaction in his brain and got him hooked on the merry-go-round of hospital admittances and toxic drugs.

His issues have still not been addressed and my son is the most loneliest person I have ever known. And I love him with my very soul. Because he has always been in my heart from the first time I looked into his dark brown eyes and held him in my arms as a new born.

And like Mary the mother of Jesus my heart has been pierced a thousand times.

Just recently despite my constant warning he felt he would be okay if he stopped taking his Depakote and wouldn't accept I had withdrawals from it myself previously last year.

I was so angry at the situation I wanted to cancel Xmas and almost did. I was angry with him for ignoring my warnings and risking what I knew would end up being another hospital admission and another addiction to medication. But I couldn't reach him.

Then the roller coaster started on it's way and he ended up delusional and walking the street at night in the wind and rain stripped to the waist and with no shoes on.

I had no choice but to call the police and they threatened to arrest me turning up with my son who was totally aggressive towards me being delusional. I was refusing to hand over my son's front door key and the female officer said a doctor couldn't be called unless I did.

So I knew the situation and had to hand it over.

He was held at the station from 2am in the morning until 11.30pm the following night. Not having slept for days properly and being totally overwhelmed and physically and emotionally exhausted.

The police told me they were waiting so long for the psychiatrist Dr. Mohamad to turn up and the allocated social worker.

To fill the forms which allow them to hand my son to a place of safety. "Safety!"

I have been witnessed to my absolute horror people dying in these places having adverse reaction to psychiatric medications. Suicidal ideation being one of the many side effects. I have been in the recovery room after my husband had ECT shock treatment and witnessed his adverse reaction to anaesthetic.

These treatments are barbaric and these psychiatrists do not apply the care for their patients by following the hipocrattic oath . Which is "First Do No Harm!" They are hypocritical.

At present I am involved via FaceBook and online with a small group of women and we are endeavouring to make a difference.

Sue Cunliffe is the daughter of a professor of medicine and she has been terribly damaged by Shock Treatment. She was a doctor and had a highly compassionate and responsible job working in a neonatal unit. Her father now retired has made huge changes for the better in his local hospital.

Jaqueline Dunn has media connections and was given Shock against her families' wishes from the age of 17 and is now brain damaged.

I know I have brain damage through being prescribed anti psychotics and the plan is I consult my GP and go for a brain scan and also be tested by a neurological psychologist for memory loss and brain impairment.

Also I am contacting my local Conservative MP who I voted for and am awaiting his reply.

In the meantime I am on my way to Manchester to visit my son and fight for his human rights. I will stay with my cousin over night and visit again the next day then make the 5 hour return journey home.

I will go to church and find support from friends there.

But most of all and the best thing I can ever do for my son is to pray to the Virgin Mother Mary and the Almighty and ever loving son of God Jesus Christ.

Anybody who reads my story and finds it of interest please do one thing for me. Please pray for us.

THE END.

www.ingramcontent.com/pod-product-compliance
Lightning Source LLC
Chambersburg PA
CBHW022155080426
42734CB00006B/439